Herbal M

Chaos in the Marketplace

Herbal Medicine
Chaos in the Marketplace

Rowena K. Richter, MPH, MBA

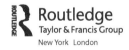

Routledge
Taylor & Francis Group
New York London

First published by

The Haworth Herbal Press, an imprint of The Haworth Press, Inc., 10 Alice Street, Binghamton, NY 13904-1580.

This edition published 2012 by Routledge

Routledge
Taylor & Francis Group
711 Third Avenue
New York, NY 10017

Routledge
Taylor & Francis Group
2 Park Square, Milton Park
Abingdon, Oxon OX14 4RN

Medicine is an ever-changing science. As new research and clinical experience broaden our knowledge, changes in treatment and drug therapy are required. While many suggestions for drug usages are made herein, the book is intended for educational purposes only, and the author, editor, and publisher do not accept liability in the event of negative consequences incurred as a result of information presented in this book. We do not claim that this information is necessarily accurate by the rigid, scientific standard applied for medical proof, and therefore make no warranty, expressed or implied, with respect to the material herein contained. Therefore the patient is urged to check the product information sheet included in the package of each drug he or she plans to administer to be certain the protocol followed is not in conflict with the manufacturer's inserts. When a discrepancy arises between these inserts and information in this book, the physician is encouraged to use his or her best professional judgment.

Cover design by Anastasia Litwak.

Library of Congress Cataloging-in-Publication Data

Richter, Rowena K.
    Herbal medicine : chaos in the marketplace / Rowena K. Richter.
        p. cm.
    Includes bibliographical references and index.
    ISBN 0-7890-1619-2 (hbk. : alk. paper) — ISBN 0-7890-1620-6 (pbk. : alk. paper)
    1. Herbs—Law and legislation—United States. 2. Herbs—Therapeutic use. I. Title.

KF1939 .R53 2002
344.73'0423—dc21

2002069076

In memory of

Varro E. Tyler

and his eloquent voice of reason
in the chaotic world of herbs

ABOUT THE AUTHOR

Rowena Richter, MPH, MBA, is currently a health policy analyst for Blue Shield of California. She is seasoned in the business, science, and regulation of herbal medicine. In 1998, she co-authored and edited a published review of European and North American herbal medicine regulations for the European Commission. (The Commission proposes new legislation to the European Union.) Prior to that, she conducted research for nearly five years at Shaman Pharmaceuticals, a start-up company that was seeking new pharmaceuticals derived from herbal medicines. She holds a master's degree in public health from the Yale School of Public Health, where she was a merit scholar, and a master's in business administration from the Yale School of Management.

Ms. Richter's thesis on the regulation of herbal medicines was selected by a panel of emeritus professors to receive the Dean's Prize for Outstanding Master's Thesis at the Yale School of Public Health in May 2000. As an undergraduate in botany in 1992, she received a national award from the American Society of Pharmacognosy for her research in natural products chemistry. She has co-authored publications in the *Journal of Ethnopharmacology* and the *Journal of Organic Chemistry*. Ms. Richter has been an invited guest lecturer on herbal medicines for a graduate course in epidemiology at the Yale School of Public Health. She has also addressed audiences of industry professionals and international scientists on the issues surrounding herbal medicine.

CONTENTS

Foreword

Dictionaries provide several definitions for the word *chaos*. It is generally used to refer to a state of utter confusion. This definition is certainly applicable to the herbal market today. However, in referring to the unorganized state of primordial matter, physicists use the word to mean a state of things where chance is the supreme determinant. This definition, too, is an apt description of the state of herbal products in the United States today.

For most consumers, chance reigns supreme when it comes to the selection of a quality botanical from the shelves of a health food store or pharmacy. Without carrying out extensive homework in advance, the bewildered would-be herbal user has absolutely no way of knowing which of the multitude of echinacea products displayed has been clinically proven to moderate cold symptoms and shorten their duration. Is the ginkgo product one that adheres to European limitations on potentially toxic ginkgolic acid, or is it one of Asian origin, which is not so regulated? Without knowing such details, including the original producer of the botanical—a fact seldom specified on the label—the consumer faces chaos.

How did the herbal situation in an otherwise developed nation such as the United States ever reach such a sad state of affairs? Rowena K. Richter's book provides in-depth answers to this perplexing question. It contains a thorough historical account of botanical regulation in this country, including an insight into the development of the most relevant current law, the Dietary Supplement Health and Education Act of 1994, commonly known as DSHEA (pronounced "duh-shay"). Everything the curious reader would like to know about this legislation—its raison d'être, the compromises involved, the final version, its enforcement, and its consequences—is covered in detail.

In addition, the book provides pertinent information on the regulation of herbal products in other developed nations, including Canada, Germany, France, and the United Kingdom. Illustrative examples of potentially useful and potentially harmful herbs are also discussed.

Other topics ranging from research and patentability to marketing, as well as several appropriate appendixes, round out the volume.

Long ago, as an academic administrator, I learned never to present a problem without offering a solution. Rowena Richter is also an advocate of that procedure. The solutions she offers are eminently sensible; they begin with the formation of an expert panel on botanicals that would categorize products on the basis of risk and evaluate the evidence on safety and efficacy, leading eventually to product quality assurance and an option to obtain drug aproval. This recommendation has been made repeatedly to the Food and Drug Administration (FDA) not only by knowledgeable individuals but also by prestigious groups such as the President's Commission on Dietary Supplement Labels. The FDA has consistently declined to act on the recommendation, citing budgetary limitations as the reason.

Personally, I view this failure to respond positively to a request that is both logical and necessary as one of the great tragedies in the health care field today. It is axiomatic that large bureaucratic agencies can almost always find money in their budgets to do what they want to do but nearly always have difficulty finding resources to do what they do not wish to do. Almost certainly, the fifty-year emphasis on drug approval of synthetic single chemical entities has played a significant role in the agency's disinterest in herbal products. Botanicals, with their multiple active principles, some of them unidentified chemically, present extremely complex problems to persons unaccustomed to dealing with them.

Somehow the Food and Drug Administration must find a way to protect and promote the health of the American people by allowing drug approval of at least certain botanicals with appropriate standards of quality. Whether it can be achieved under the rules set forth in August 2000 by the FDA in its guidance document for the botanical drug products industry is still problematic.

No herb has attained drug approval in recent times under either of the two routes (over-the-counter monograph expansion or investigational new drug/new drug application) described therein. Until one has received approval, it is uncertain just how much data will be required to support a successful application. In the meantime, it is my hope and belief that this useful volume detailing the history and current status of botanical regulations in this country as well as in other developed nations will facilitate the process of drug approval and the establishment of quality standards for botanical medicines in the United States.

Varro E. Tyler, PhD, ScD, Dr. rer. nat.
(1926-2001)
Distinguished Professor Emeritus
Purdue University, W. Lafayette, Indiana

Preface

American consumers have driven each major policy change since the United States began regulating food and drugs in 1906. The Dietary Supplement Health and Education Act of 1994 (DSHEA) is no exception. DSHEA ushered in a new era for herbal medicines. Since 1994, these products have proliferated in the United States and so, too, has the number of Americans consuming them.

People around the world have used herbal medicines since the beginning of civilization. Yet regulating herbal medicines in the modern age has proved to be an enormous challenge. Consumers want to benefit from access to quality herbal products and at the same time be protected from the associated risks.

This book began as my master's thesis at the Yale School of Public Health. I set out to evaluate the situation of herbal medicines in the United States from a public health perspective. The supplement industry, the FDA, and the media have each taken a stand on the issue. I wanted to focus on what the regulations and resulting marketplace mean for the health of American consumers. Why and how has the United States wound up classifying herbal medicines alongside vitamins and minerals as dietary supplements, a subcategory of food? The rest of the industrialized world views herbal medicines as drugs, in some cases distinguishing them from pharmaceuticals. What are the implications of this choice for American public health in terms of both benefits and risks? As it turned out, in May 2000, I won the Dean's Prize for Outstanding Master's Thesis in Public Health.

The reader will see influences from my background in science, industry, and policy. As an undergraduate I studied botany and natural products chemistry. As a professional, I researched aboriginal herbal medicines for their pharmaceutical potential. As a graduate student, I explored the role of policy in the herbal medicine marketplace and co-authored and edited a regulatory review for the European Commission.

Herbal medicines have the potential to contribute positively to the health of Americans, as they have for generations around the world. However, in the United States we are falling short with these products both in promoting and protecting public health. In this book, I attempt to take a levelheaded look at where we are with herbal medicines, how we got here, and where we need to go to improve matters for the American people.

Acknowledgments

The information presented in this book could not have been compiled without the generous assistance of many people from many countries. I would like to thank my faculty advisor at the Yale School of Public Health, Lowell Levin, for introducing me to the Association of the European Self-Medication Industry (AESGP) through which I found an extraordinary opportunity to collaborate on a regulatory review for the European Commission. Through this experience and the resulting document I was able to study the regulation of botanicals in Europe. I am grateful to my colleagues in Brussels: Hubertus Cranz, Barbara Steinhoff, Jean-François Dechamp, and Johan Lindberg; in Canada: David Skinner, Grace Chaves, Bruce Erickson, Frank Chandler, and Cathy Airth; and in the United States: Marilyn Barrett.

I would also like to express my appreciation to my thesis readers at the Yale School of Public Health. Each brought his or her own valuable expertise in public health to bear on this multifaceted topic: Nora Groce from medical anthropology and international health; John Thomas from a health policy, legal, and regulatory viewpoint; and Susan Mayne from the perspective of chronic disease epidemiology.

Finally, I thank the entire team at The Haworth Herbal Press for all their guidance and expertise, and Marty Jezer for his indexing talents.

I wish to gratefully acknowledge all of these individuals for their contributions. Any errors, omissions, and opinions are my own.

PART I:
INTRODUCTION

Chapter 1

Overview

The use of herbal medicine* in the United States has increased dramatically over the past decade. In 1990, only 2.5 percent of American adults had used at least one herbal medicine in the previous twelve months. By 1997, this figure had risen to 12.1 percent, and Americans were spending $5.1 billion out of pocket for herbal medicines.[1] In 1999, sales began to plateau and remained flat in 2000. However, in a period of just five years herbal medicine products had become as widely available to consumers as vitamins. They are now found in supermarkets, pharmacies, and numerous other mainstream retail outlets. Botanical medicines, similar to all pharmacologically active substances, have the potential to contribute positively, neutrally, or negatively to the health status of the American population. This book argues that the current regulatory and business environment constrains both the potential health benefits and the protection from risk.

Part I frames the problem with two brief examples. Part II begins by reviewing the pertinent U.S. regulatory history. Next, to place the U.S. situation in an international context, Part II considers the regulations in Canada, Germany, France, and the United Kingdom. From this comparison, common themes as well as variations emerge. The three European countries were selected because they have some of the most highly evolved regulations for herbal medicines. Canada is included because it is currently revamping its regulations and has thought

---

*In this book, the terms *botanical, botanical medicine, herbal medicine, herbal product,* and *phytomedicine* are considered equivalent. In the United States, botanicals are considered the subcategory of food known as dietary supplements and are not considered drugs, with a handful of exceptions. However, because (a) people generally consume botanicals with the intention of addressing a particular health condition; and (b) the rest of the industrialized world regulates botanicals as drugs, the term *herbal medicine* will be used in this book.

3

through the issues in an exemplary fashion. Each nation's approach is specific to its politics, history, and culture, and the United States would not and should not simply copy them. However, the experience of these other industrialized countries does inform the analysis of the U.S. situation. Part III illustrates practical implications of the U.S. regulations with six examples. The first three illustrations demonstrate how herbal medicines could contribute more to public health. Indeed, two of these botanicals have captured the attention of the National Institutes of Health (NIH) and warranted multimillion-dollar clinical trials. The second set of examples highlights the public health risks associated with the current situation. Part IV analyzes the public health issues related to safety, research, clinical practice, consumer interests, business, media, and federal government. Part V offers a few key, high-impact recommendations.

THE DILEMMA

The public health problem represented by botanicals in the current U.S. regulatory and business environment is framed here with two examples. One situation is potentially beneficial; the other is potentially harmful.

St. John's wort (*Hypericum perforatum* L.) was the first botanical selected by the National Institutes of Health (NIH) to be the subject of a clinical trial. The NIH study was largely motivated by a meta-analysis published in the *British Medical Journal* in 1996. That study of 23 randomized clinical trials concluded that St. John's wort may be useful for treating mild to moderate depression, is superior to placebo, and has fewer side effects than pharmaceutical antidepressants. Soon after, in October 1997, the NIH began a 3-year, $4.3 million, multi-center clinical trial on St. John's wort. However, rather than selecting patients with mild to moderate depression to participate in the study, NIH chose patients with moderately severe depression and found both St. John's wort and Zoloft (a best-selling pharmaceutical antidepressant) to be ineffective treatments in this trial. In their report in the *Journal of the American Medical Association,* the researchers noted that "Hypericum may be most effective in less severe major depression . . ." and this possibility remains an open question in the United States. In Germany, however, St. John's wort products are commonly prescribed and widely studied. So far in the United States, consumers cannot even be certain that what is on the label will be in the bottle of any herbal medicine they purchase.

In contrast, the potential risks of ephedra (also known as ma huang) have raised widespread public health concerns because ephedra products contain ephedrine alkaloids. Two billion doses of botanical ephedrine alkaloids are consumed in the United States annually. Among herbal products, the U.S. Food and Drug Administration (FDA) most frequently receives adverse event reports for products containing ephedrine alkaloids. Based on these reports and the scientific literature, in June 1997 the FDA issued a proposed rule to limit the allowable dose of ephedrine alkaloids in botanical products to 8 mg per serving.[3] However, in July 1999 the U.S. General Accounting Office (GAO) issued its response to the FDA's proposed rule.[4] It questioned the basis for the FDA's conclusions about causation and the proposed dose. The GAO pointed out that even by the FDA's own account, the passive adverse event reports that the FDA cited often lacked information on product identification, doses ingested, duration of use, and medical diagnoses. The scientific data on dosage of ephedrine alkaloids is also incomplete. The FDA's final rule is pending. Meanwhile, legislation on ephedra has been proposed independently in several states (Texas, California, Indiana, Virginia, Vermont, Illinois, Hawaii, Iowa, New York, New Hampshire, Montana, Pennsylvania, and Massachusetts). Proposals range from complete bans on ephedra (in Texas, which was rejected) to exemptions for restrictions of over-the-counter sales of botanical ephedrine products (in Montana). The National Football League, the National Collegiate Athletic Association, and the International Olympic Committee have each banned ephedrine use.

PURPOSE OF THIS BOOK

The public health objectives that are guiding the analysis of botanicals in this book are: (1) to minimize the risk of adverse events (i.e., first do no harm); (2) to enhance the population-wide benefits of the potential favorable contributions (including potential cost savings in some cases, such as with St. John's wort); and (3) to seek ways to develop and provide incentives for a system that allows distinctions to be made among herbal products and treatments on a sound, scientific basis.

PART II:
REVIEW OF REGULATIONS

Chapter 2

United States

HISTORY OF REGULATION OF BOTANICALS

According to David Kessler, former head of the Food and Drug Administration (FDA), "regulating supplements that people take for medicinal purposes is one of the most difficult issues for the Food and Drug Administration over the last century."[1] This section provides a historical context. First, it summarizes the evolution of U.S. regulations that pertained to botanicals prior to 1990. Second, it analyzes the politics of the process that led to the Dietary Supplement Health and Education Act (DSHEA) of 1994. DSHEA, as mentioned, currently governs herbal medicines in the United States.

Regulations Pertaining to Herbal Medicines Prior to 1990

Overview

Many of the herbal medicines that are currently on the market were already in use when the United States began regulating food and drugs in 1906. For that reason, many herbs have been grandfathered from one statute to the next and have been exempted from requirements to prove safety and efficacy for most of U.S. regulatory history. As will be evident from the summary in this section, they have also escaped labeling restrictions until recently.

Pure Food and Drugs Act of 1906

This act was the first U.S. statute to regulate interstate commerce of domestically manufactured food and drug products.[2] It established minimal standards for quality, purity, and strength, but it did not address safety or efficacy. Under this act the regulating agency had to show deliberate fraud to establish a violation.[3] This act was repealed and replaced with the Federal Food, Drug, and Cosmetic Act of 1938.

Sherley Amendment of 1912

This amendment, passed by the U.S. Congress, added labeling regulations to the Pure Food and Drugs Act of 1906. Fraudulent or false claims of therapeutic effects of medications were termed "misbranding" for the first time.[4]

Federal Food, Drug, and Cosmetic Act of 1938

In 1937, seventy-three people died after ingesting Elixir Sulfanilamide, which contained diethylene glycol (also known as antifreeze).[5] Under the 1906 Act,[6] premarket testing of the elixir had not been required. In response to this tragedy, the U.S. Congress passed the Federal Food, Drug, and Cosmetic Act of 1938 (FDC Act). The FDC Act, similar to the Pure Food and Drugs Act of 1906, still focused on safety, adulteration, and misbranding. It gave the FDA new authority to test a drug for safety in humans and to determine whether a food or drug was safe, even in the absence of fraud. The FDC Act also established the FDA's powers of criminal prosecution, injunction, and seizure.[7] For new drugs, the FDC Act required proof of safety and submission of a new drug application (NDA). This statute, with its subsequent amendments, currently regulates food and drugs in the United States.

Drug Amendments of 1962

From 1938 until 1962, the FDA was only authorized to regulate drugs when marketing approval was sought, which was generally after human clinical trials had already been conducted to establish safety.[8] After the thalidomide tragedy* in Europe and Canada, the public in the United States demanded tighter drug regulation. In re-

---

*Thalidomide was introduced in West Germany on October 1, 1957. Between 1957 and 1961, it was marketed in Europe, Japan, Australia, and Canada as a treatment for symptoms of morning sickness in pregnant women. As a result, thousands of children were born with severe birth defects. Thalidomide was withdrawn from the market in 1961 and 1962.

sponse, the U.S. Congress in 1962 amended the FDC Act[9] to shift the burden of proof for both safety and efficacy onto manufacturers, thereby eliminating automatic approval of new drug applications. The 1962 Amendment required manufacturers to prove efficacy in addition to safety prior to marketing a drug. Manufacturers were then also required to obtain FDA approval before conducting the necessary "adequate and well-controlled" clinical investigations to demonstrate efficacy.[10]

Botanicals tend to be natural ("works of nature") or generic products without substantial human innovation involved, which makes patenting difficult.[11] The fact that botanicals often contain complex mixtures of compounds also complicates patenting. Without patent protection, the U.S. herb industry lacks an incentive to invest in expensive research on the safety and efficacy of their products.

Review of Over-the-Counter Drugs
Begins in 1972

When it was enacted in 1938, the FDC Act required proof of safety and submission of an NDA for new drugs. In 1962, the FDC Act was amended to also require proof of efficacy for new drugs. The FDA then undertook a review of all drugs that had been approved for marketing between 1938 and 1962 on the basis of safety data alone. In 1972, FDA established the OTC Drug Monograph Review system[12] and began reviewing the safety and efficacy of all OTC drugs that either were not covered by an NDA or were approved prior to 1962 solely on the basis of safety data.

This review was conducted on approximately 100,000 OTC drugs that were on the market in 1972 to bring them into compliance with the 1962 Amendment standards for safety and efficacy. Because of the huge number of drugs requiring OTC review, the FDA established seventeen panels of experts by therapeutic class. Each panel investigated active drug constituents rather than individual products. OTC monographs were then published on drug classes and categorized by therapeutic effect, thereby establishing doses of active ingredients considered generally safe and effective.[13] The results of the OTC review were first released to the public in 1990. The OTC Drug Review Program is ongoing.

Many botanicals and other products that were marketed before 1938 had been grandfathered into the FDC Act of 1938 under the Pure Food and Drugs Act of 1906, and therefore had previously been exempt from proving safety and efficacy. Since the OTC review in 1972, botanicals cannot be marketed as OTC drugs unless they qualify as either "old drugs" or "new drugs." In either case, the botanical must be generally recognized as safe and effective (GRASE) in accordance with the OTC monographs. In addition, old drugs must have been marketed in the United States to a material extent and for a material time; until January 2002, foreign marketing experience was not considered. New drugs must have an approved NDA. Few botanicals have retained their OTC status as old drugs* and so far none have been approved as new drugs through an NDA.[14] As discussed later in this chapter, difficulties with patenting, multiple active ingredients, and the exclusion of foreign (particularly European) market experience from material extent and material time have all played a role in limiting the number of botanicals approved as OTC drugs in the United States to date.

Classification of Botanicals Becomes More Ambiguous

As herbal medicines were squeezed out of the OTC category, another classification for them was needed. At this point in regulatory history, botanicals could still be considered food additives. Disagreement ensued between the FDA and manufacturers about which category was most appropriate for botanicals. For food additives, the burden of proving safety falls on the manufacturer. Not surprisingly, the FDA favored food additive status for botanicals. In contrast, for foods, the FDA bears the burden of proving the product is dangerous to the public health. Manufacturers of botanicals therefore preferred to classify their products as dietary supplements (a subcategory of food). As dietary supplements, botanicals were regulated under the amended Recommended Daily Allowance (RDA) statute of 1976 (also known as the Proxmire Amendment of 1976). This amendment permitted dosing information on dietary supplement labels for the first time. However, no label claims could be made regarding effects on bodily struc-

---

*These are primarily laxatives, such as psyllium, cascara, and senna. Pure OTC compounds that have been derived from botanicals are generally not considered to be herbal medicines.

ture or function, or curing, preventing, or mitigating disease.[15] The Proxmire Amendment of 1976 also restricted the FDA's powers to limit the potency of vitamins and minerals and prohibited regulation of dietary supplements as drugs.

Public Awareness of the Link
Between Nutrition and Health

As consumer interest in nutrition grew, manufacturers responded by making nutritional claims about their food products. Some firms began advertising the value of their products in preventing or treating various diseases. Between 1978 and 1990, "in response to public concerns regarding potential inaccurate or misleading claims by manufacturers,"[16] the FDA proposed several amendments to the Food, Drug, and Cosmetic Act. Although the amendments were defeated, this effort reflected "a growing awareness of the role that nutrition plays in health. . . . 'The American public wants better nutrition information,' said Rep. Henry A. Waxman (D-California), chairman of the Energy and Commerce Subcommittee on Health and the Environment. 'But when consumers try to look beyond the marketing hype displayed on food packaging and investigate the actual nutrition content of a product, they are greeted with a bewildering array of contradictory and misleading information.' "[17] Consumer groups continued to demand that Congress take action to police the labeling and advertising claims.[18] The result was the Nutrition Labeling and Education Act of 1990.

Nutrition Labeling and Education Act
(NLEA) of 1990

This act[19] was passed by Congress in response to demand from some (but not all) consumer organizations for the FDA to address the proliferation of health-related claims on nondrug products.[20] NLEA primarily required labeling of foods with content of fat, cholesterol, sodium, carbohydrates, sugar, protein, and dietary fiber. Under NLEA, premarket FDA approval would be required for health claims made on supplement labels and for safety. This legislation also exempted supplement products, including herbs, from "new drug" classification. The herb and dietary supplement industries felt very threatened by the passage of the NLEA and the labeling restrictions of the earlier Proxmire Amendment, and they began to fight vigorously for their rights. Notably, the NLEA had been opposed by Senator Orrin Hatch (R-Utah) among others. Senator Hatch's concern was that the bill would result in "higher food prices and more and more government intrusion in American lives."[21]

Political Analysis of the Dietary Supplement Health and Education Act

This section analyzes the agenda setting, problem definition, and legislative process that culminated with the Dietary Supplement Health and Education Act of 1994 (DSHEA). The FDC Act as amended by DSHEA regulates nearly all botanicals sold on the U.S. market today.

Senator Hatch's Agenda

The single most important event that placed dietary supplements on the national agenda was initiated by Senator Hatch in 1992. It occurred when David Kessler, then head of the FDA (and a former Hatch staff member) was pushing an unrelated bill through Congress that would require prescription drug manufacturers to pay "user fees" to help offset the cost of federal safety and efficacy reviews. Hatch was the ranking Republican on the Senate Labor and Human Resources Committee and an important player in the creation of FDA policy. Hatch had been a longtime supporter of Kessler's user fee concept. In a Senate hearing at the very end of the 102nd Congress, however, Hatch sought to delay Kessler's bill. Hatch said that he did not see a need for immediate action on the user fee bill. During the heated debate between Kessler and Hatch that ensued, Hatch tied in an unrelated issue. He brought up his amendment that would "place a one-year moratorium on implementation of nutrition labeling regulations as they applied to food supplements such as vitamins and herbs. Kessler, noting that he was speaking for himself and not for the administration, said he might be amenable to such a moratorium. The admission was something of a surprise, because the FDA chief had gained national acclaim—and managed to outrage both the food and drug industries—with his unrelenting attacks on questionable health claims."[22] Hatch's political maneuver was successful. The Hatch amendment on dietary supplements was soon after signed into law, buried as Title II in the Prescription Drug Fees Provisions (PL 102-571).

The Hatch agenda gained momentum from that point on. Hatch's motivation behind the amendment was fairly clear: dietary supplements were an important industry in Utah (generating over $1 billion in sales annually)[23] and he personally was an avid user of vitamins and herbs. His primary agenda was probably to fend off the stricter, more established food and drug regulations for his industry friends in Utah (some of whom were his former staff members) for as long as possible. They had built up their industry during two decades of relaxed regulations and would fight hard to hold onto their corner of the market. (During his attempt at a presidential campaign in 2000, Hatch repeatedly boasted that he had saved the supplement industry with DSHEA.[24]) Serving industry interests well, in addition to delaying labeling regulations, the amendment ordered studies of the regulations of other countries on health claims and temporarily barred the FDA from disapproving U.S. health claims for dietary supplements.

Supplement Manufacturers and Their Consumer Coalitions

Groups representing the supplement manufacturers had been outraged by the FDA's authority to regulate label claims through NLEA and later dubbed Senator Hatch "our man of the year."[25] They argued that NLEA (without the Hatch amendment) would put them out of business. Groups such as the Council for Responsible Nutrition, Citizens for Health, Nutritional Health Alliance, National Nutritional Foods Association, Utah Natural Products Alliance (representing eight major Utah-based dietary supplement manufacturers), and ACT UP (AIDS activists) began to rally their membership together in support of the dietary supplement manufacturing industry with statements such as, "The FDA is using [the regulations] as a way to take products off the market."[26]* Dramatic protests were staged with

---

*This quote is reprinted with permission from the October 7, 1994, edition of *Legal Times* © 1997 NLP IP Company. All rights reserved. Further duplication without permission is prohibited.

black ribbons, "blackout" days, petitions and letter campaigns to senators,[27] and a CompuServe computer bulletin board called "Holistic Health Forum,"[28] all driven by the fear that the FDA was working to shut down the dietary supplements industry.[29] " 'This is the No. 1 mail issue' in Congress, [said] Anthony Podesta, president of the Podesta Associates lobbying firm. 'More than the crime bill, more than health care, more than the budget.' "[30]*

FDA Position

Brad Stone, a press spokesperson for the FDA, responded to consumer fears with the following statement.

> While it's true there's been some legitimate disagreement about what the standard should be for health claims, what isn't true are some of the wild allegations being made that somehow FDA is going to remove a whole group of dietary supplements from the market or that we're going to make them by prescription only or that we're going to limit the potency. All that stuff is just a bunch of nonsense. In fact, not only have we not proposed that [limiting the potency], but we couldn't do it even if we wanted to. There's a law preventing us from doing that [Proxmire Amendment of 1976].[31]

Consumer Groups

Meanwhile, other consumer groups supported the FDA, saying "Hatch's approach would unleash a public-policy disaster. The bill, they [said], weakens FDA's ability to protect consumers from fraudulent supplement manufacturers while granting carte blanche to the industry to make outrageous, unscientific claims regarding the value of its products."[32]* John Gleason of the Center for Science in the Public Interest said the Hatch bill "just doesn't cut it when you're trying to summarize highly technical scientific information for the benefit of consumers. . . . The kind of information these labels contain is not

---

*This quote is reprinted with permission from the October 7, 1994, edition of *Legal Times* © 1997 NLP IP Company. All rights reserved. Further duplication without permission is prohibited.

verifiable by consumers. You just can't conduct a double-blinded, randomized, clinical trial in your basement."[33]*

Consumer groups in this camp included the American Association of Retired Persons (AARP), American Cancer Society, American Heart Association, and Consumers Union. Jo Reed, AARP's senior coordinator for consumer issues, asserted that supplement industry supporters "were very effective in mobilizing people based on false and misleading information."[34]* These consumer groups supported an alternative bill introduced by Representative Cardiss Collins (D-Illinois) which would "foster the use of beneficial supplements by permitting well-founded health claims and leave harmless, honestly labeled supplements alone. It would also ensure that supplements actually contain what they claim."[35] Henry A. Waxman (D-California) was Chairman of the Energy and Commerce Subcommittee on Health and the Environment and would oppose the Hatch bill, as would Energy and Commerce Committee Chairman John D. Dingell (D-Michigan).

Discussion of Agenda Setting

As the stakeholders and their opposing agendas solidified, it became apparent that the divisions were not along party lines and unusual alliances, such as that between Senator Hatch and ACT UP, were forming. Despite wide-ranging positions, there was consensus among all camps on two points. First, that consumer access to dietary supplements should be maintained. Second, that consumers needed—indeed, were demanding—better information about dietary supplements. The controversy swirled around how to define what "better" information should be. It was generally agreed that the information consumers wanted about health-related effects of dietary supplements was "scientific" information. However, there was bitter disagreement over who should conduct the research, who should pay for the research, who should interpret the results, what constituted a scientifically valid health claim, and whether dietary supplements should be presumed safe or unsafe.

Hatch and his supporters insisted that consumers should have unlimited access to the scientific literature as part of the marketing of

---

*This quote is reprinted with permission from the October 7, 1994, edition of *Legal Times* © 1997 NLP IP Company. All rights reserved. Further duplication without permission is prohibited.

herbal products (and dietary supplements in general). With this approach consumers would interpret the scientific findings themselves, which Hatch touted as a First Amendment right. Hatch was also clear that the FDA should be responsible for any testing required to dispute health claims. Hatch was essentially attempting to maintain the status quo for as long as possible.

Hatch's opponents had less consensus on their position, which probably limited their effectiveness. They were strongest in advocating FDA approval of specific health claims for dietary supplements. However, their argument was weakened because it was based partially in the drug classification and partially in the food classification. On one hand, they referred to drugs by maintaining that the public is no more capable of interpreting the scientific literature on dietary supplements than they are the literature on prescription or OTC drugs. On the other hand, they referred to food by arguing that there should not be a double standard between food safety and dietary supplement safety. Hatch's clear unambiguous designation of dietary supplements as a distinct category was very strategic for his agenda. It introduced an array of complex and cumbersome issues for the FDA and required the huge bureaucracy to nimbly and quickly rethink safety, efficacy, labeling, and enforcement in the face of massive consumer support for the supplement industry.

Legislative History of DSHEA

As a result of the political process, the Hatch agenda was later compromised, but nonetheless it began a new era in the regulation of herbal medicines and dietary supplements. The remainder of this section examines the modifications made to the Dietary Supplement Health and Education Act of 1994 (DSHEA) as it proceeded through the 102nd, 103rd, and 104th Congresses. By this time dietary supplements represented a $4-billion market and were used by approximately half of all Americans.[36] The perception of the problem at hand ranged from access for consumers to public health hazards. With Clinton's health care revisions on the presidential agenda, the "problem stream" and "political stream" converged to create a window of policy opportunity that was quickly seized by both sides of the dietary supplements debate.[37]

DSHEA was at the heart of the heated controversy over the appropriate role of the state in regulating the supplement industry. Sentiments reflecting both the nonresponsiveness of the bureaucracy and the legitimacy of the bureaucracy would powerfully influence the debate.[38] The public would flood their congressional leaders with letters of support for DSHEA and express their fears about the intrusion of the state into their rights. In David Kessler's words, "Americans view their government with a mixture of reliance and mistrust. We want to be free to choose whatever products we like until something goes wrong. Then we turn to our government and want to know why it happened and what the government is doing about it."[39] Even opposing sides agreed that the overarching goals were rational regulation of dietary supplements, freedom of choice for consumers, access to truthful information, and protection and enhancement of public health. There was also consensus among all stakeholders that dietary supplements are playing an increasingly important role in American public health. This discussion focuses on the most contentious aspects of the legislation: access to information on dietary supplements; standards of scientific evidence; FDA enforcement rights; and the burden of proving safety. To clarify the development of these key issues, the discussion begins with the 102nd Congress.

102nd Congress (1992): Hatch Squares Off Against the FDA

Senator Orrin Hatch (R-Utah) seized the opportunity[40] to represent industry interests by maneuvering his dietary supplements amendment onto the agenda during the 102nd Congress. The Dietary Supplement Act was signed into law on October 29, 1992, in the form of Title II of the unrelated Prescription Drug Fees Provision (PL 102-571). With conservative Hatch as the Senate sponsor and liberal Representative Bill Richardson (D-New Mexico) teaming up as the House sponsor, it was clearly a bipartisan, bicameral issue. Hatch made his position clear when he said, "It is not Democrat vs. Republican; it is the United States Congress vs. the Food and Drug Administration."[41]

Substance of PL 102-571

This measure essentially bought time for Hatch's agenda. It delayed the application of the NLEA to dietary supplements with a one-year moratorium through December 15, 1993. Furthermore, it guaranteed the issue would be revisited during the 103rd Congress by requiring promulgation of new regulations for dietary supplements by June 15, 1993, and finalization of the new regulations by December 31, 1993. The following issues were put on the table with PL 102-571 and served as the starting place for discussions during the 103rd Congress:

Access to Information About Dietary Supplements. The Health and Human Services (HHS) secretary could approve health claims for supplement labels during the moratorium.

Standard of Scientific Evidence. The health claims for labels could be approved only if there was "significant scientific agreement" about the claims.[42] This standard is the same one applied to foods such as breakfast cereal and orange juice under NLEA.

FDA Enforcement Rights. Hatch did all he could to put the FDA on the defensive with regard to its dietary supplement enforcement activities. PL 102-571 required that the General Accounting Office (GAO) issue a report (due one year later, with an interim report due after six months) examining the FDA's use of resources for regulation of dietary supplements. (The GAO found that the FDA had no particular plan to target the supplement industry and was responding as needed to consumer complaints and information about health risks.)[43] The measure also required that the Office of Technology Assessment write a report (due within six months) investigating the relationship between the regulation of dietary supplements and health outcomes; emphasis was to be placed on the regulatory approaches of other countries.

Burden of Proving Safety. For the moment, this issue was overshadowed by the inquiry into FDA practices.

*FDA Cracks Down on Supplement Retailers
and Manufacturers*

The FDA did not adopt a defensive posture. Early in 1993, the FDA tried to ban the sale of black currant oil capsules based on an animal study that linked one of the components in the oil to brain seizures. The FDA claimed that the oil was a food additive that was added to the gelatin capsule (the food). Two federal appeals courts (Seventh Circuit and First Circuit) overruled the FDA, characterizing their legal arguent as an irrational "Alice-in-Wonderland approach."[44,45,46]* During the debates in the 103rd Congress, Hatch supporters would frequently cite this case as evidence of the FDA's regulatory excesses and would use it to fuel the public's fear that the FDA was going to take their vitamins away unless Congress took action.

103rd Congress of 1993

Senator Hatch introduced the Dietary Supplement Health and Education Act (DSHEA) to the 103rd Congress on April 7, 1993, as S 784. Representative Bill Richardson (D-New Mexico) introduced a similar bill in the House as HR 1709. The bills were proposed as an amendment to the Federal Food, Drug, and Cosmetic Act. The most controversial points were as follows:

Access to Information About Dietary Supplements. The bills sought to loosen the restrictions over the health claims permitted on supplement labels (creating exemptions from NLEA).

Standard of Scientific Evidence. The FDA had been using the strictest standard for health claims on labels under NLEA: "significant scientific agreement."[47] The Hatch legislation, in response to the "FDA's lack of enthusiasm for the product they are regulating,"[48] proposed to lower the standard to "significant scientific evidence."[49]

FDA Enforcement Rights. The Hatch bill did not increase FDA authority to remove unsafe supplement products from the market because FDA already had "ample authority."

Burden of Proving Safety. The FDA would be responsible for disproving product safety.

Interest groups fell into two strong lobbying camps. Industry representatives and consumers supported the Hatch bill and demanded continued access to dietary supplement products and information. They were quick to point out the regulatory excesses of the FDA (e.g., citing the black currant oil capsules). Some feared that if the FDA got its way, they would have to "kiss [their] vitamins good-

---

bye."[50] Opponents of the Hatch bill were concerned about the excesses of some (not all) supplement manufacturers in the form of unsafe ingredients and outrageous health claims (particularly regarding botanicals and amino acids). Their goal was to keep the FDA involved in the regulation of label claims and premarket safety approval.[51] In May 1993, President Clinton expressed his support for the Hatch bill and welcomed dietary supplements in discussions about health care.[52]

FDA Advance Notice of Proposed Rulemaking

In response to the Dietary Supplement Act of 1992, the FDA issued a report on June 18, 1993. It announced the FDA's position on the regulation of dietary supplements.[53] The FDA proposed to restrict allowable health claims to those supported by significant scientific agreement, cap the potency of vitamins and minerals (countering the Proxmire Amendment of 1976), treat certain herbs as drugs or food additives, and classify amino acids as prescription drugs.[54] With this report, the two poles of the debate were firmly established.

List of Unsubstantiated Claims Issued by the FDA

Hatch then requested HHS to provide a list of dietary supplement products that contained false or misleading health claims and for which the FDA lacked authority to halt marketing. In response, HHS issued a list of 243 products made by 114 companies. Hatch staff members then selected a sample of five companies from the list to investigate. Hatch says they found

> that not only had each company been notified by FDA of its concern, but also that each company had removed the health claim questioned by FDA. I came away from this examination with three conclusions. First, FDA does have the authority to act on supplements that pose a problem. Second, the industry is generally responsive to FDA. And third, FDA is reluctant to admit it.[55]

With this maneuver, Hatch eroded the FDA's credibility regarding its current regulatory efforts on dietary supplements and made the ground more fertile for compromise.

House Subcommittee on Health and the Environment, Committee on Energy and Commerce, July 29, 1993

Both Hatch and FDA Commissioner David Kessler gave statements at this hearing. Kessler said, "In the absence of a clear standard, the best FDA can do to try to separate the good from the bad when it comes to supplements is to go after these products one by one."[56] He also made it clear that the FDA did not have the resources to pursue all cases, only the most urgent ones, with the caveat that 80 percent of nutritional supplements (i.e., most vitamins and minerals) on the market pose no regulatory problems. He went on to say, "Freedom of choice means little unless consumers have . . . accurate information."[57] He then presented a report listing 500 unsubstantiated health claims made by supplement manufacturers and associated actions taken by the FDA. The report also included adverse events associated with sixteen ingredients being sold as components of dietary supplements. The report further described how undercover FDA agents had visited 129 health food stores nationwide and posed as customers asking for cures for infections, high blood pressure, or cancer. The agents were apparently advised to take a variety of supplements.[58,59] "FDA Targets Untrue Product Claims" was the headline in *The Washington Post* the next day.[60]

Safety Concerns

Dramatizing the FDA's concern about the hazards of supplements, Dorothy Wilson, who suffered from eosinophilia myalgia syndrome (EMS), testified before the subcommittee from her wheelchair about L-tryptophan. This amino acid was once commonly prescribed by physicians for insomnia and anxiety. It has since been linked to forty deaths and over 1,000 injuries from severe muscle pain and paralysis associated with EMS.[61] Ms. Wilson said she had assumed L-tryptophan was safe because it was prescribed by her doctor. Committee Chairman John D. Dingell (D-Michigan), in a surprise appearance before the subcommittee, pointed out that without sufficient regulatory authority the FDA has to wait until problems with supplements occur before it can take action. He also invoked the thalidomide scandal.[62] After such a heart-rending personal testimony from Ms. Wilson, backed by the committee chairman, it became difficult for Hatch to make a case that the FDA's ability to address such threats to public health should be limited, and safety concerns remained central to the debate.

In promoting his bill, Hatch used his own dramatic effects to support his argument. He invoked the First Amendment right for consumers to have access to scientific information on supplements. Using the tragic story of folic acid and the prevention of neural tube defects (NTDs) and spina bifida, Hatch was quick to point out that the CDC recommended the use of folic acid in 1991, the HHS made the same recommendation in 1992, but the FDA did not approve this label claim until 1994 after a public outcry (and "some 100 babies a month [had been born] with NTDs that could have been prevented with folic acid"). In June 1994 he published an article entitled, "Congress versus the Food and Drug Administration: How One Government Health Agency Harms the Public Health." Strengthening ties to Clinton's reforms, Hatch also asserted that access to dietary supplements would help to lower health care costs.[63]

Public Protests

On August 12, 1993, health food stores around the country placed black shrouds over some of their dietary supplement displays to dramatize industry concerns about the pending FDA regulations and in support of Hatch's and Richardson's bills.[64] The massive letter-writing campaigns and public interest in DSHEA began to make blocking the bill politically unwise for elected officials.

Senate Committee on Labor and Human Resources,
October 21, 1993

Committee Chairman Edward M. Kennedy (D-Massachusetts) opposed the Hatch bill and submitted an alternative. Kennedy's version prohibited marketing supplements that presented a "reasonable possibility of harm."[65] It gave the FDA more regulatory powers than the Hatch bill, which allowed FDA action only if a supplement presented a "substantial and unreasonable" risk of harm.[66] Hatch (the ranking Republican on the committee) and Kennedy were unable to reach a compromise. However, Hatch did modify his bill as follows:

Standard of Scientific Evidence. Rather than "significant scientific agreement" (FDA's wording) or "significant scientific evidence" (Hatch's previous language), the standard in the latest version of the Hatch bill was changed. Health claims could appear on supplement labels unless the FDA found that the "totality of scientific evidence" indicated the claim was invalid.[67] Products that had been on the market for years without negative health effects would have been considered safe for use.[68]

On November 17, 1993, the Hatch bill (S 784) was shelved. Kennedy proposed a compromise bill (S 1762) that would buy time until April 15, 1994. The Senate passed S 1762 by voice vote on November 20, 1993, and it was sent to the House Energy and Commerce Committee the next day. However, the House did not approve S 1762 before the end of the year, which meant the moratorium was over and FDA could put the full NLEA regulations in place in the spring of 1994.[69]

Another Alternative Bill Fails

During the 103rd Congress, Representative Cardiss Collins (D-Illinois) had introduced alternative legislation as the Dietary Supplement Consumer Protection Act, which applied the same standards used for regulation of food. The bill was aiming to deliver "what the Hatch/Richardson bills promise—without the special-interest exemption from honest labeling."[70] Their concern was that under the Hatch bill the results of a study could be printed on a label even if the study was "preliminary, irrelevant for humans [i.e., conducted in animals or in vitro] or never confirmed"[71] and would leave consumers to interpret scientific data. The Collins bill was supported by many organizations such as Consumers Union, the American Heart Association, and the American Cancer Society but failed to out-compete the Hatch bill.[72]

104th Congress (1994): Senate Committee on Labor and Human Resources

S 784 (DSHEA) was approved (12-5) by the Senate Committee on Labor and Human Resources on May 11, 1994. The decision was hailed as a victory for supplement manufacturers. Kennedy's substitute was rejected (5-12). However, several significant changes from Hatch's original bill were made at the last minute:

New Definition of Dietary Supplements. The final bill set a broad statutory definition of dietary supplements. The new definition would prevent the FDA from regulating dietary supplements as either drugs or food additives. Kennedy remained concerned that the broad definition, especially the inclusion of "botanical extracts" as dietary supplements, might create regulatory loopholes that would allow foreign drugs into the U.S. market without FDA approval.[73]

Access to Information About Dietary Supplements. Hatch made a major concession to opponents in an attempt to resolve the contentious issue of health claims on supplement labels. Recognizing that Congress lacked the expertise needed to settle the question, he moved the issue out of the legislative arena and into the executive branch. Hatch's bill mandated a two-year presidential commission to develop guidelines for health claims on dietary supplement products. The commission would have seven members with "expertise and experience in dietary supplements and in the manufacture, regulation, distribution and use of such supplements."[74] The bill (S 784) also stipulated "no member of the commission shall be biased against dietary supplements."[75] Meanwhile, the FDA could restrict the kinds of information that stores were permitted to display near supplement products and prohibit labels that linked product ingredients with healthy body function.[76]

Standard of Scientific Evidence. Hatch also conceded that while the executive label commission did its work, the FDA could continue to prohibit manufacturers from making health claims unless there was significant scientific agreement to support them. This standard was established for foods by the 1990 Nutrition Labeling and Education Act (PL 101-535).[77] To further address this issue and again move the debate outside the legislative forum, the bill called for establishment of the Office of Dietary Supplements within the National Institutes of Health. This office would be mandated "to promote scientific study of the benefits of dietary supplements in maintaining health and preventing chronic disease and other health-related conditions."[78]

Burden of Proving Safety and FDA Enforcement Rights. The FDA would be required to prove a product is unsafe, if used as directed, before being able to pull the supplement off the market.[79]

Debate on the Floor of the House and Senate

The amended Hatch bill (S 784) was passed by the Senate on August 13, 1994, by unanimous voice vote. The final round of amendments took place in the House in long negotiations between Hatch (who wanted "to relax existing labeling rules on the grounds that they were burdensome") and Dingell and Waxman (who were "concerned about preserving the power of the Food and Drug Administration (FDA) to regulate the supplements").[80] The final version of S 784 was passed by the House on October 7, 1994, by voice vote. The same bill was passed by the Senate later that same day. The final modifications represented considerable concessions by Hatch:

Access to Information About Dietary Supplements. Health claims on labels would follow FDA standards for four (not two) more years while the seven-member independent commission decided on labeling regulations and HHS adjusted the rules. In addition, manufacturers could use this disclaimer on labels to protect themselves: "This statement has not been evaluated by the Food and Drug Administration. This product is not intended to diagnose, treat, cure or prevent any disease." As Hatch wanted, stores were permitted to display information on supplements from sources other than the manufacturers, provided the information was not "false or misleading." The final wording describing the seven commissioners was that they "shall be without bias on the issue of dietary supplements."[81]

FDA Enforcement Rights. The FDA was permitted to pull a product off the market if it could provide evidence that the product caused a "significant or unreasonable risk" of illness or injury. This standard was lower than the "substantial and unreasonable" standard required in the previous versions by Hatch.[82]

Burden of Proving Safety. Supplements could continue to be sold without premarket FDA approval. However, manufacturers were required to submit evidence that new products were safe seventy-five days before marketing, and the FDA was permitted to block marketing if the evidence was not satisfactory (this aspect is closer to the food additive generally recognized as safe (GRAS) status provisions[83]).[84]

Conclusion

DSHEA was signed into law by President Clinton on October 25, 1994. Neither side was completely satisfied, but both sides supported the final version. The supplement industry viewed the outcome of DSHEA quite favorably:

> When it enacted the Dietary Supplement Health and Education Act of 1994, Congress recognized the role supplements can play in health promotion and in the prevention of chronic diseases such as cancer, heart disease, and osteoporosis. This comprehensive piece of legislation established a new regulatory framework for supplements, ensuring continued access to safe products, made to quality standards. It also allowed for increased dissemination of information about the health benefits of these products.[85]

In contrast, critics of DSHEA continued to say it is "bad public policy and a sellout to the industry's marketing ambitions."[86]* They pointed out that

> Even the most well-informed, health-conscious individual would be hard-pressed to assess the reliability of health claims based on animal studies, clinical-intervention trials or epidemiological studies. . . . Health claims based on preliminary scientific studies are misleading, and the Supreme Court has stated firmly that such "commercial speech" can be prohibited by consumer-protection agencies. . . . As a recent editorial in the *New England Journal of Medicine* recognized, such studies are meant to guide further scientific research, not used as the basis for public-health recommendations.[87] (Reprinted with permission of *Insight.* Copyright 2002 News World Communications, Inc. All rights reserved.)

---

*This quote is reprinted with permission from the October 7, 1994, edition of *Legal Times* © 1997 NLP IP Company. All rights reserved. Further duplication without permission is prohibited.

DSHEA left nutraceuticals and "functional foods" (i.e., foods eaten expressly for their nutritive content) in a legal gray area. That market segment has expanded enormously in the regulatory vacuum since 1994.[88] A congressional bill addressing nutraceuticals was introduced on October 1, 1999. It is discussed later in this chapter.

Only two DSHEA provisions received funding: the Presidential Commission on Dietary Supplement Labels and the Office of Dietary Supplements. However, Congress appropriated only $1 million for the latter out of the $5 million authorized by DSHEA. Other DSHEA provisions were not funded at all, such as the Office of General Counsel review of FDA's Generally Recognized as Safe list to bring it into compliance with DSHEA and the Center for Food Safety and Applied Nutrition. The President's Commission on Dietary Supplement Labels issued their report in November 1997 and was then disbanded. Their report is discussed in more detail later.

DSHEA was born out of an opportunity to create policy during which negotiations and compromises were possible in part because Hatch and Kessler were comparable in clout and political savvy. The resulting statute has ushered in a new era in the regulation of dietary supplements at a time when raising the health status of Americans is a top priority for the federal government. With the supplement market growing at record rates, the full impact of this legislation remains to be seen.

CURRENT LEGAL CLASSIFICATION OF BOTANICALS

Depending upon their intended use, herbal products may be defined as foods (e.g., fruits, vegetables, teas, spices, or flavorings), dietary supplements (a subcategory of food), drugs, or cosmetics. So-called functional foods and nutraceuticals are not legally defined and may be sold as either foods or dietary supplements, depending upon the intended use of the product. Legislation that proposed to address nutraceuticals is discussed later in this chapter. Cosmetics are not considered in this book.

Dietary Supplement Status

Dietary supplement status (which is legally in the classification of food) is by far the most common choice made by manufacturers for their herbal products to date, since no premarket approval is required. The definition of the term "dietary supplement" was established in Section 3 of the Dietary Supplement Health and Education Act of 1994 (DSHEA),[89] which amended Section 201 of the Federal Food, Drug, and Cosmetic Act with 21 U.S.C. 321 (ff). Dietary supplements include products that are intended to supplement the diet and contain a vitamin; a mineral; an herb or other botanical; an amino acid; a dietary substance for human use to supplement the diet by increasing the total dietary intake; or a concentrate, metabolite, constituent, extract, or combination of any of these ingredients. Dietary supplements must be labeled as such and do not include tobacco, food products that are marketed as conventional foods, or products that are represented as the sole item of a meal or the diet. Note, however, that a dietary supplement may be sold in conventional food form. Thus an herbal tea can be either a conventional food or a dietary supplement, depending upon the intended use of the product. In the *Federal Register* dated April 22, 1996, the Food and Drug Administration (FDA) clarified that under the existing statute dietary supplements are for use by humans and therefore DSHEA does not apply to products intended for animal (nonhuman) use. This stipulation contrasts with drugs, which can be intended for human or animal use.

Disease claims, express or implied, are not permitted for dietary supplements. Under the FDC Act, a product intended to diagnose, treat, cure, mitigate, or prevent any disease is considered a drug. DSHEA does allow statements of nutritional support in the labeling of dietary supplements that describe general well-being or the intended effect on the structure or function of the human body. These statements are commonly known as "structure/function claims." In the *Federal Register* dated April 29, 1998, the FDA issued a proposed rule further distinguishing "structure/function claims" from "disease claims." The FDA received 235,000 comments on their proposed rule and held a public meeting on August 4, 1999, to further discuss the most controversial issues. On January 6, 2000, the FDA released its final rule. This topic is discussed further under Structure/Function Claims.

DSHEA explicitly excludes dietary ingredients intended for use in a dietary supplement from the definition of "food additive." This means that Section 409 of the FDC Act is not applicable to such ingredients. The term "food additive" is defined in Section 201(s) (21 U.S.C. 321(s)). For food additives, the burden of proving safety falls on the manufacturer. In contrast, for foods, the FDA bears the burden of proving that the product is dangerous to the public health.

Under DSHEA, articles that have been approved as new drugs, certified antibiotics, and licensed biologics are excluded from the definition of dietary supplement. Also excluded are articles authorized for investigation as new drugs, antibiotics, and licensed biologics for which substantial clinical investigations have become publicly known. These exclusions apply if the article was not marketed as a dietary supplement or food prior to such approval or authorization (and clinical investigation).

The interpretation of this DSHEA provision was the basis for a recent legal case. The litigation centered on the interpretation of DSHEA with regard to marketing of an herbal product (Cholestin) which contains a naturally occurring compound (mevinolin). In April 1997, the FDA asserted to the manufacturer of Cholestin that mevinolin is chemically indistinguishable from lovastatin. Lovastatin was approved in 1987 by the FDA as a new drug for lowering cholesterol under the brand name Mevacor. Under DSHEA, articles that have been approved as new drugs are excluded from the definition of dietary supplement if the article was not marketed as a dietary supplement or food prior to the new drug approval. On this basis, on May 20, 1998, the FDA announced that it would ban the import of red yeast rice (*Monascus purpurea* Went., the raw material for Cholestin) from China.[90] A subsequent injunction permitted the manufacturer of Cholestin to import the specific quantities of red yeast rice needed to meet sales predictions.[91]

The FDA's position in this suit implied that because Cholestin contains a constituent which has been approved as a new drug, Cholestin is also considered to be a drug and not a dietary supplement. One key to the interpretation of DSHEA in this case was whether the fact that the compound lovastatin is present in the herbal product may be used in the marketing and labeling of the herbal product. This case raised complex legal issues. More specifically, it set precedent for interpreting what is meant by the relevant "article" for purposes of Section 321(ff)(3)(B)(i) of DSHEA. This section excludes "an article that is approved as a new drug" from the definition of dietary supplement. The Cholestin case hinged on whether the "article" refers to a finished drug product (Mevacor) or to the active ingredient contained therein (lovastatin). The manufacturer of Cholestin (Pharmanex) asserted that neither lovastatin nor Cholestin should be considered such an "article" because they have not been approved as finished drug products. Pharmanex supported its argument with citations of FDA regulations, Supreme Court decisions, lower court decisions, and an FDA administrative decision.[92] On February 16, 1999, after reviewing the scientific, medical, and legal evidence, the Federal District Court of Utah reversed the import ban and upheld the original classification of Cholestin as a dietary supplement rather than a drug.[93] The court sustained Pharmanex's position "both because they show[ed] that FDA has consistently fought to advance it and because this Court must assume that Congress acted with the knowledge of such pre-existing authorities."[94] The FDA appealed the Utah judge's decision.[95]

On July 21, 2000, the United States Court of Appeals for the 10th Circuit reversed the United States District Court's decision and sent the case back to that court for review of specific questions related to the records. On March 30, 2001, the U.S. District Court issued a Memorandum Decision and Order affirming that Cholestin is a drug—not a dietary supplement. The Court concluded that red yeast rice products that contain lovastatin are unapproved drugs and their sale as dietary supplements is prohibited on that basis. However, because lovastatin only occurs in red yeast rice that has been fermented, the FDA maintains that red yeast rice products that do not contain lovastatin (or other substances approved as drugs) may be sold as dietary supplements.[97]

Over-the-Counter Drug Status

Under the FDC Act, a product intended to diagnose, treat, cure, mitigate, or prevent any disease is considered a drug. In practice, few (if any) U.S. manufacturers market their botanicals as OTC drugs. In principle, botanicals can attain over-the-counter (OTC) drug status in either of two ways: (1) monograph system: as an "old drug" by being grandfathered from the Pure Food and Drugs Act of 1906 into the FDC Act of 1938, and subsequently being approved by inclusion as a new active ingredient in an OTC monograph through the OTC Drug Monograph Review program; or (2) new drug approval system: as a "new drug" by receiving approval through a new drug application (NDA). Very few botanicals have retained OTC status through the OTC Drug Monograph Review program. Of the botanical ingredients that were included in the OTC review, six were listed as safe and effective for their intended uses (e.g., cascara bark, senna leaf, and psyllium seed as laxatives) and over 150 were eliminated from the review process or were found to be unsafe, ineffective, or lacking sufficient evidence for evaluation.[97] To date, no botanicals have been approved as new OTC drugs through the new drug application process, although several applications are in progress. There is increasing industry interest in the botanical OTC market segment as the profits and the demand for quality herbal medicines grow, but the following requirements have defeated all attempts so far.

Standards of Safety and Efficacy

In all cases, to attain OTC drug status a product must be generally recognized as safe and effective (GRASE) in accordance with federal regulations.[98] Under current regulations, safety can be established based on published studies in some cases, but acute and long-term animal toxicological studies may also be required. Proof of efficacy generally demands double-blinded, placebo-controlled human clinical trials to meet the requirement of adequate and well-controlled studies.[99]

Patent Protection

Since substantial research is required to obtain OTC status, the issue of patent protection is relevant here. Because botanicals tend to lack substantial human innovation[100] and often contain complex mixtures of compounds, patenting is difficult (but still possible). Manufacturers have had insufficient market incentive to patent and conduct extensive research on their herbal products for two reasons: (1) the results would also be available to their competitors; and (2) herbal products can be marketed as dietary supplements without these substantial investments in research.

Single Active Constituents

The drug approval process is designed for pharmaceuticals that typically contain one active ingredient. Botanicals frequently have multiple active ingredients, which further complicates the approval process. Under current regulations, manufacturers have been required to demonstrate the safety and efficacy of each ingredient in a combination cocktail, an insurmountable hurdle.

Material Extent and Material Time

A substance is considered an old drug (i.e., it does not require an NDA) if it meets two conditions: (1) it is GRASE and (2) it has been marketed to a "material extent" and for a "material time" for a particular OTC indication.[101] Until 2002, the FDA based material extent and material time on marketing experience in the United States. This interpretation was maintained by convention and is not explicitly stated in the FDC Act. For botanicals, this interpretation of the law is particularly significant because much of the experience with the most popular herbal medicines on the U.S. market comes from Europe.

In 1992, the European-American Phytomedicines Coalition (EAPC) submitted two citizen petitions for herbal products (for valerian as a sleep aide and for ginger as an antiemetic or for relief of symptoms of motion sickness). In their petitions they requested that the FDA amend its policy with regard to evaluation of substances for inclusion in the OTC Drug Monograph Review system by permitting use of foreign data. In response to the EAPC petitions and seven other petitions on this issue, the FDA published an advance notice of proposed rulemaking (ANPRM) on October 3, 1996, clarifying their position on the use of foreign data and marketing experience and inviting public comment.

The FDA issued its proposed rule[102] on December 20, 1999, followed by a comment period, and its final rule[103] on January 23, 2002. This change lowers what has been one of the major barriers to botanical OTC drugs in the United States. It provides a procedure for submitting a time and extent application (TEA) that may demonstrate marketing "for a material time" and "to a material extent" based on U.S. or *foreign* experience. The data must span a minimum of five continuous years in at least one country. If marketing involved more than five countries, the TEA is required to include information from the five countries with the longest and most extensive experience. Once the TEA is approved, as a second step, manufacturers would submit safety and efficacy data. It remains to be seen how achievable the TEA standards will be in practice.

Presidential Commission's Recommendations
on Botanicals as OTC Drugs

In November 1997 the President's Commission on Dietary Supplement Labels reviewed eighteen regulatory schemes from other countries and the World Health Organization. It concluded that twelve of the eighteen allow a more streamlined means of approving therapeutic claims for botanicals labeled as drugs and recommended that "a comprehensive evaluation of regulatory systems used in other countries for botanical remedies is needed."[104] The Commission did not conduct such a study themselves because it was beyond their mandate.

The Commission made it clear that they were not recommending that dietary supplement status be changed from foods to drugs. However, it did conclude that "more study is needed regarding the establishment of some alternative system for regulating botanical products that are used for purposes other than to supplement the diet but that cannot meet OTC drug requirements."[105] It also strongly recommended that the FDA "promptly establish a review panel for OTC claims for botanical products that are proposed by manufacturers for drug uses."[106] It stated that "Botanicals have always been included as potential candidates for OTC status. The Commission is not recommending a new category of OTC drugs, but believes that a dedicated OTC panel on botanicals would facilitate the review of appropriate OTC claims."[107] The Commission observed that the uses of dietary supplements are sometimes similar to those of OTC drugs and noted that "in some cases, there is current scientific evidence to support such use [for prevention or treatment purposes]."[108]

FDA's Response to the Presidential Commission's Report

In the *Federal Register* of April 29, 1998, the FDA responded that it does not have adequate resources to conduct a full study of how botanical products are regulated around the world. However, the FDA also indicated that it intended to issue a proposed rule addressing the Commission's suggestion that certain botanicals be treated under the OTC Drug Monograph Review system.

FDA released its guidance for industry[109] on August 11, 2000, and accepted comments until March 15, 2001. Its final rule is expected during 2002. Once finalized, these changes could be a substantial breakthrough for OTC botanicals in the United States. They address what have been some of the biggest roadblocks for OTC approval of botanicals as previously described (standards of safety and efficacy, patent protection, and multiple active constituents). The guidance lays out the criteria for botanical drug approval through OTC monographs, new drug applications (NDAs), and initial drug applications (INDs), including clinical investigations. (An NDA is required when the drug is not generally recognized as safe and effective. Before conducting clinical trials in support of an NDA, an IND is needed.)

Some of the key features of the new policies are the following:

- The guidance "discusses several areas in which, because of the unique nature of botanicals, FDA finds it appropriate to apply regulatory policies that differ from those applied to synthetic, semisynthetic, or otherwise highly purified or chemically modified drugs (including antibiotics)."[110]
- Reduced requirements for preclinical safety, chemistry, manufacturing, and controls for botanicals that have been legally marketed in the United States as dietary supplements or cosmetics without any known safety concerns.
- An exemption from the requirements for combination drugs. A botanical drug with multiple constituents can be tested as one drug, provided a single formulation is used and its composition remains constant.
- An OTC monograph application must comply with an existing *United States Pharmacopeia* monograph or propose a new one.
- OTC monograph status that any manufacturer can utilize.

- NDA drug status that provides a period of exclusivity, during which no other manufacturer can apply for the same approval or submit an OTC monograph application for the same product. For products with no patent, the exclusivity period is three years. With a patent, the exclusivity periods lasts five years.

Once this guidance is finalized, the next landmark would be actual approval of OTC botanicals through each of these routes.

Homeopathic Drug Status

Under the FDC Act, articles listed in the *Homeopathic Pharmacopoeia of the United States* are legally defined as drugs. When the FDC Act was passed in 1938, such articles were essentially grandfathered into the definition of a drug. However, drugs listed in the *Homeopathic Pharmacopoeia of the United States* continue to be exempt from premarket FDA review of safety and efficacy. Products that are sold as homeopathic remedies must comply with the specifications set out in the *Homeopathic Pharmacopoeia of the United States* and relevant regulations. A homeopathic drug product may not contain any nonhomeopathic active ingredients and therefore is rarely formulated in combination with dietary supplements.

CURRENT REGULATION
AND SURVEILLANCE OF BOTANICALS

Overview

The Federal Food, Drug, and Cosmetic Act of 1938 as subsequently amended governs the marketing and sale of food, drugs, and cosmetics in interstate commerce in the United States, including those dispensed by a practitioner. The Food and Drug Administration (FDA) is primarily responsible for interpreting and enforcing the FDC Act. In principle, herbal products that will be marketed with disease claims are considered drugs and are currently subject to the drug provisions of the FDC Act. In practice, most botanicals are sold as dietary supplements, which are regulated by the FDC Act as amended by the Dietary Supplement Health and Education Act of 1994 (DSHEA). Advertising of botanicals in all media is governed by the

Federal Trade Commission Act[111] and the Federal Trade Commission's criteria for support of food advertising claims.[112,113] Each state is responsible for locally produced and marketed herbal products that do not enter interstate commerce. There are no laws specific to the origin of the botanical.

Well-Known Botanicals

Dietary supplement ingredients that were marketed before October 15, 1994, are considered to be safe unless the FDA demonstrates otherwise. FDA's list of botanical ingredients that are generally recognized as safe (GRAS) includes essential oils, extracts, spices, and flavorings for use in foods, and natural flavoring agents for use in foods and beverages.

New Dietary Ingredients

Dietary supplement ingredients that were first marketed in the United States after October 15, 1994, are defined by Section 8 of DSHEA as new dietary ingredients. A dietary supplement product that contains a new dietary ingredient is deemed adulterated unless it meets one of two conditions: (1) either it must be an ingredient that has previously been in the food supply in the same chemical form; or (2) the manufacturer must submit evidence for the conclusion that there is a reasonable expectation that the new dietary ingredient will be safe when it is used under the conditions recommended on the label. The supporting information may include published scientific studies, a history of use, previous presence in the food supply, or other evidence that establishes the safety of the herbal product. Scientific publications used as evidence must be fully cited. In contrast to OTC drugs, in principle a history of safe use is considered valid evidence for purposes of establishing the safety of new dietary ingredients. In practice, it remains to be seen whether data on historical use alone will be sufficient to conclude that a new dietary ingredient can "reasonably be expected to be safe" as required by DSHEA.

DSHEA requires the manufacturer to submit all evidence at least seventy-five days before the new dietary ingredient enters interstate commerce. The FDA estimates that a company will spend twenty hours extracting and summarizing the necessary data from its files;[114]

industry did not dispute this estimate.[115] The FDA may prohibit marketing if not satisfied with the evidence, but premarket authorization is not required. Ninety days after receipt, the FDA must place the nonproprietary information provided by the manufacturer on public display.

Scientific Standards

Issues relating to scientific standards, the effectiveness of products, and the dissemination of information regarding health-related benefits of dietary supplements have posed considerable regulatory challenges for industry, the FDA, and state regulatory agencies. Following are detailed discussions of the regulatory situation.

Section 485C of DSHEA mandated the establishment of an Office of Dietary Supplements within the National Institutes of Health. Under DSHEA, this office was mandated to: (1) conduct and coordinate scientific research; (2) collect and compile results of scientific research; and (3) serve as the principal advisor to other government agencies on issues relating to dietary supplements. However, in practice this office has received limited funding and FDA has continued to play the primary role in regulating dietary supplements. The President's Commission on Dietary Supplement Labels recommended that the Office of Dietary Supplements be funded at the level authorized by DSHEA and place greater emphasis on its advisory role. The Commission also suggested that the supplement industry establish an expert advisory committee to guide it on technical issues, particularly related to labeling. Labeling standards are discussed later in this chapter.

Manufacturing Standards

Control of Raw Material

The existing Current Good Manufacturing Practice (CGMP) regulations for food, which also apply to dietary supplements, allow certification from the supplier of the raw material in lieu of direct testing by the manufacturer of the finished product. In the *Federal Register* of February 6, 1997, the FDA requested comments on the adequacy of such certification for dietary supplements, particularly for lesser known ingredients. The FDA's final rule on this issue is pending.

Control of Raw Material from Foreign Sources

The FDA is mandated to ensure the safety of the nation's food supply by the Federal Food, Drug, and Cosmetic Act and the Public Health Service Act.[116] As part of that mandate, FDA conducts Good Manufacturing Practices (GMP) inspections in the United States and its territories. In practice, inspections in foreign countries are conducted infrequently. However, issues regarding imported dietary supplements and dietary ingredients remain on the agenda for GMP discussions. With regard to exporting botanicals, there is a distinction made from products that are intended for sale within the United States. The FDA Export Reform and Enhancement Act of 1996[117] allows the import of certain components of dietary supplements for further processing only if the final product is intended for export.[118]

Control of Intermediate Products

DSHEA regulations apply both to dietary supplements and to ingredients intended for use in a dietary supplement. The Current Good Manufacturing Practices for dietary supplements that were proposed in 1997 also cover intermediate products or "dietary ingredients" intended for use in the manufacture of dietary supplement finished products.

Good Manufacturing Practices

In November 1994, Section 9 of DSHEA extended the application of existing GMP regulations[119] to include dietary supplements. Dietary supplement products are required to be prepared, packaged, and stored in accordance with Current Good Manufacturing Practices (CGMP) applicable to food products. All ingredients must be truthfully and accurately listed on the label and the product may not be adulterated with other substances. Section 9 of DSHEA also gave the option to develop GMP regulations specifically for dietary supplements, modeled after CGMP regulations for food and not imposing standards for which there is no current and generally available analytical methodology.

In November 1995, draft CGMP regulations were submitted to the FDA by representatives of the dietary supplement industry. The industry draft was modeled after GMP regulations for foods, with additional provisions specific to dietary supplements as needed. In particular, "there [was] no desire or intent to impose on dietary supplements the type of documentation and validation currently required in the manufacture of pharmaceutical products."[120] The FDA reviewed the draft and issued it as a proposed rule in the *Federal Register* of February 6, 1997, opening a comment period to address specific questions. Among the issues raised by the FDA were the following: whether regulations are needed and, if they are needed, whether they should be mandatory or voluntary; the appropriateness of applying defect action levels for foods (i.e., spices and flavorings) to dietary supplements given the differences in consumer exposure levels; procedures for positive identification of botanical dietary ingredients; the need for documentation of day-to-day quality control procedures for dietary supplements (these would be beyond the requirements for foods); the involvement of competent medical authorities (in addition to quality control personnel) in the evaluation of adverse event reports; the need to specify procedures for evaluating the seriousness of adverse event reports; the need for evaluation and documentation of the safety of dietary supplements; and quality control of computer software programs and equipment used in GMP procedures.

Finally, the FDA suggested that the principles of Hazard Analysis and Critical Control Points (HACCP) might be more appropriate and less burdensome than the regulatory approach submitted by industry. The inspection procedure now used evaluates the conditions at the time of inspection but does not assess the adequacy of ongoing food safety assurance programs within a company. In contrast, with an HACCP system food processors assess the hazards specific to their products, use routine controls to prevent or minimize those hazards, monitor the performance of the controls, and maintain regular records. To make their inspections more preventive of (rather than reactive to) food safety problems, the FDA has proposed incorporating HACCP into the food inspection regulations, which would also govern dietary supplements.

The public comment period on these issues ended on June 6, 1997. The FDA's Good Manufacturing Practices for Dietary Supplements Working Group of the Food Advisory Committee held a public meeting on October 16, 1998, "to further develop a draft report on good manufacturing practices identity testing and recordkeeping."[121] On

July 12, 1999, the FDA held the first in what was intended to be a series of public meetings to "understand the economic impact that any proposal to establish Current Good Manufacturing Practices (CGMP) regulations for dietary supplements may have on small businesses in the dietary supplement industry."[122] Topics included "manufacturing practices and standard operating procedures for: (1) personnel, (2) buildings and facilities, (3) equipment, (4) lab operations, (5) production and process controls, and (6) warehousing, distribution and post-distribution of raw, intermediate and final products"[123] and "a discussion about the verification of the identity, purity, and composition of dietary supplements and dietary supplement ingredients."[124]

DSHEA mandated in 1994 that good manufacturing practices be established for botanicals. In February 2002, more than seven years later, FDA reported[125] that it plans to issue a proposed rule for dietary supplement GMPs by the middle of FY 2002, followed by a ninety-day comment period, review of comments received, and a final rule during FY 2003.

Labeling

The Presidential Commission on Dietary Supplement Labels

During the legislative debates that led up to DSHEA, U.S. Congress was unable to resolve some of the technical issues concerning the appropriate use of labeling and accompanying literature for dietary supplements. Instead they deferred to outside expertise, and DSHEA mandated the presidential appointment of a seven-member Commission on Dietary Supplement Labels within the executive branch. The Commission was authorized by DSHEA to "evaluate how best to provide truthful, scientifically valid, and not misleading information to consumers. . . ."[126] Members of the Commission were appointed by President Clinton on November 9, 1995, and given two years to complete their assignment. They submitted their report[127] to the president, U.S. Congress, and the secretary of Health and Human Services in November 1997.

The Commission was mandated to issue its "recommendations" as proposed rules that could be opened for public comment, revised, and then become regulations. They also chose to add two other categories of conclusions that would not be considered proposed rules: Findings and Policy Guidance. "Findings" were simply conclusions. "Policy Guidance" was advice to agencies, groups, or individuals but was not intended as proposed rules for lawmaking. The Commission's report incorporated the testimonies and input of hundreds of individuals from the general public, from the supplement, food, and drug industries, from the scientific community, from health professions, consumer groups, and from federal and state agencies.[128]

Structure/Function Claims

DSHEA restricts nutritional support claims made on dietary supplement labels to descriptions of "the role of a nutrient or dietary ingredient intended to affect the structure or function in humans"[129] or "the documented mechanism by which [the supplement] acts to maintain such structure or function."[130] Nutritional support claims, preferably called structure/function claims, must be accompanied by the following disclaimer: "This statement has not been evaluated by the Food and Drug Administration. This product is not intended to diagnose, treat, cure, or prevent any disease." Prior to DSHEA, making a structure/function claim on a label would have rendered that product a drug. Consequently, since DSHEA was enacted there has been considerable regulatory ambiguity in the distinction between "disease claims" and "structure/function claims." To address this need for clarification, the specific criteria that distinguish a disease claim from a structure/function claim were published by the FDA in the *Federal Register* as a proposed rule on April 29, 1998[131] (see Tables 2.1 and 2.2). In that publication, the FDA also requested comments on "the distinction between *maintaining normal function,* which is potentially the basis for an allowable structure/function claim, and *preventing or treating abnormal function,* which is potentially a disease claim . . . and on factors that help distinguish between claims relating to normal, healthy function that do not imply disease treatment or prevention and those that do"[132] [emphasis added]. The FDA issued its final rule on January 6, 2000.[133] The revisions are shown in Table 2.1. Table 2.2 summarizes rejection rates for claims. Table 2.3 shows examples of acceptable structure/function claims and implied disease claims under the latest FDA rules.

TABLE 2.1. FDA's Proposed Criteria for Distinguishing Disease Claims from Structure/Function Claims

Disease Claim Criteria	Examples of Disease Claims
1 An effect on a specific disease or class of diseases	"protective against the development of cancer" (structure/function: "helps promote urinary tract health")
2 Reference to a set of signs or symptoms in scientific or lay terminology that are recognizable as characteristic of a specific disease or diseases	"improves urine flow in men over 50 years old"—characteristic of benign prostatic hypertrophy (structure/function: "improves absentmindedness")
3 References to certain natural states that are not diseases themselves but are associated with abnormalities which are characterized by a specific set of signs and symptoms and therefore fit the proposed definition of disease	premenstrual syndrome, hot flashes, Alzheimer's disease, decreased sexual function associated with aging
Revised in final rule: Common conditions associated with natural states or processes that do not cause significant or permanent harm will not be treated as diseases. . . . Uncommon or serious conditions . . . will continue to be treated as diseases	*Revised in final rule:* Disease claims include senile dementia, toxemia of pregnancy, severe depression associated with the menstrual cycle, cystic acne (structure/function: hot flashes, common symptoms associated with the menstrual cycle, ordinary morning sickness associated with pregnancy, mild memory problems associated with aging, hair loss associated with aging, noncystic acne)
4 Labeling that suggests expressly or implicitly that the product will diagnose, cure, mitigate, treat, or prevent disease: (a) product name; (b) statements about the formulation, including a claim that the product contains an ingredient that has been regulated by the FDA as a drug and is well-known to consumers; (c) reference to citations with a disease name in the title; (d) use of the word "disease" or "diseases"; (e) suggesting an effect through pictures, vignettes, symbols, or other means	(a) "Hepatacure"—liver problems (structure/function: "Cardiohealth" or "Heart Tabs"); (b) aspirin, digoxin; (c) "Serial Coronary Angiographic Evidence that Antioxidant Vitamin Intake Reduces Progression of Coronary Artery Atherosclerosis"; (e) electrocardiogram tracings, pictures of organs, Rx symbol
(c) *revised in final rule:* the use in labeling of a publication title that refers to a disease will be considered a disease claim only if, in context, it implies that the product may be used to diagnose, treat, mitigate, cure, or prevent disease	(c) *revised in final rule:* highlighting, bolding, using large type size, or prominent placement of a citation that refers to a disease use in the title; placing a citation to a scientific reference that refers to a disease in the title on the immediate product label or packaging

5 Reference to certain product classes that are strongly associated with the diagnosis, cure, mitigation, treatment, or prevention of a disease or diseases — antibiotic, laxative, analgesic, antiviral, diuretic, antimicrobial, antiseptic, antidepressant, vaccine (structure/function: energizer, rejuvenative, revitalizer, adaptogen)

6 Stating the effect is similar to that of a recognized drug or therapy. Suggesting use as an adjunct to a recognized drug or disease therapy — "Herbal Prozac"; "use as part of your diet when taking insulin to help maintain a healthy blood sugar level" (structure/function: "use as part of your weight loss plan")

7 Claiming to augment the body's own disease-fighting capabilities, either to a disease or to the vector of a disease — "supports the body's antiviral capabilities"; "supports the body's ability to resist infection" (structure/function: "supports the immune system")

8 Claiming to counter the adverse events resulting from medical intervention — "reduces nausea associated with chemotherapy"; "helps avoid diarrhea associated with chemotherapy" (structure/function: "helps maintain healthy intestinal flora")

9 Otherwise suggesting an effect on a disease or class of diseases

Source: Food and Drug Administration. 1998. Regulations on statements made for dietary supplements concerning the effect of the product on the structure or function of the body. *Federal Register* 63(82):23624-23632.

TABLE 2.2. FDA Rejection Rate for Common Structure/Function Claims

Type of Claim	Total Submissions	Percent Rejected	Number Rejected
Cholesterol, cardiovascular health, circulation	170	27	46
Joint and arthritis	120	26	31
Cold, allergy, and infection	150	25	37
Digestion	145	19	27
Antioxidant and immune system	160	14	22
Improve mental health and promote relaxation	270	4	10
Increase energy, vitality, or stamina	200	2	4

Source: Adapted from the Tan Sheet. *F-D-C Reports.* October 5, 1998.

TABLE 2.3. Acceptable Structure/Function Claims and Unacceptable Implied Disease Claims

Acceptable Structure/Function Claims	Unacceptable Implied Disease Claims
Helps to maintain cholesterol levels that are already within the normal range	Lowers cholesterol
Supports the immune system	Supports the body's antiviral capabilities
Helps support cartilage and joint function	Reference to helping "joint pain"
Maintains healthy lung function	Maintains healthy lungs in smokers
Arouses or increases sexual desire and improves sexual performance	Helps restore sexual vigor, potency, and performance
For the relief of occasional sleeplessness	Helps to reduce difficulty falling asleep

Source: Adams, Chris. Splitting hairs on supplement claims: Under the FDA's guidelines, improving health is ok; curing a disease isn't. *The Wall Street Journal.* February 22, 2000.

Reprinted by permission of *The Wall Street Journal*, Copyright © 2000 Dow Jones & Company, Inc. All Rights Reserved Worldwide. License number 245520477121.

The comment period for the original proposed rule was extended until September 28, 1998, and the FDA received over 100,000 comments. On July 8, 1999, the FDA announced a public meeting would be held on August 4, 1999, to discuss three of the most contentious issues that had arisen over structure/function claims. The comment period was also reopened until August 4, 1999.[134] The three most controversial issues that were raised through comments are:

(1) Whether FDA should retain the definition of "disease or health-related condition" issued for NLEA health claims, rather than issue a new definition of "disease"; (2) whether certain common conditions associated with natural states, such as hot flashes associated with menopause, or premenstrual syndrome associated with the menstrual cycle, should be considered "dis-

eases"; and (3) whether dietary supplements may carry implied disease claims.[135]

The summarized comments on these three issues follow.

Definition of disease. Existing federal regulations[136] issued in 1993 to implement the health claims provisions in NLEA defined a "disease or health-related condition" as:

> damage to an organ, part, structure or system of the body such that it does not function properly (e.g., cardiovascular disease), or a state of health leading to such dysfunctioning (e.g., hypertension); except that diseases resulting from essential nutrient deficiencies (e.g., scurvy, pellagra) are not included in this definition.[137]

However, the FDA did not use this definition in their proposed rule of April 29, 1998, "because its use of the term 'damage' could be interpreted to limit the definition to serious or long-term diseases, and might exclude conditions that are medically understood to be diseases, such as depression and migraine headaches."[138] Instead, the FDA proposed the following new definition of disease on April 29, 1998:

> any deviation from, impairment of, or interruption of the normal structure or function of any part, organ, or system (or combination thereof) of the body that is manifested by a characteristic set of one or more signs or symptoms (including laboratory or clinical measurements that are characteristic of a disease).[139]

According to the FDA, the dietary supplement industry and individuals favor the NLEA definition, commenting that the new definition is too broad and tends to include many minor conditions that are not diseases. Health professional groups, on the other hand, support the new definition because of its consistency with the medical definition of disease. In the FDA's final rule issued on January 6, 2000,[140] it deleted its proposed definition and adopted the NLEA definition of a disease or health-related condition.

Common conditions associated with natural states. The FDA's proposed rule of April 29, 1998, treats a condition as a disease when it presents "a characteristic set of signs or symptoms recognizable to health care professionals or consumers" as an "abnormality."[141] The FDA's examples of such conditions include toxemia of pregnancy, premenstrual syndrome, hot flashes, decreased sexual function associated with aging, and Alzheimer's disease. No comments disputed the fact that toxemia of pregnancy and Alzheimer's are diseases. However, many comments asserted that premenstrual syndrome, hot flashes, and decreased sexual function associated with aging are so common that they should not be treated as abnormal or as diseases. In the final rule of January 6, 2000, the FDA revised this criterion as follows:

> Common conditions associated with natural states or processes that do not cause significant or permanent harm will not be treated as diseases under the final rule. For example, hot flashes, common symptoms associated with the menstrual cycle, ordinary morning sickness associated with pregnancy, mild memory problems associated with aging, hair loss associated with aging, and noncystic acne will not be treated as diseases under this provision. Uncommon or serious conditions like senile dementia, toxemia of pregnancy, severe depression associated with the menstrual cycle, and cystic acne will continue to be treated as diseases under the final rule.[142]

The inclusion of morning sickness on this list of allowable structure/function claims set off public health alarms. Several experts pointed out the risks for pregnant women and their fetuses. They reminded the FDA that it had protected U.S. women by not approving thalidomide and urged it to reconsider its position on dietary supplement claims for morning sickness.[143] The FDA responded immediately (within a week) by advising supplement manufacturers not to make any label claims related to pregnancy.[144] The FDA plans to publish a *Federal Register* notice, hold a public meeting, then issue further guidance on the issue of label claims related to pregnancy. They are working to overcome this significant public health blunder.

Implied disease claims. "Express disease claims" are those claims that mention the name of the disease and are undisputedly considered to be disease claims. "Implied disease claims" do not mention the name of the disease explicitly. The FDA proposed to treat implied disease claims as disease claims, too. As such, these claims would require premarket FDA approval either as health claims or drug claims. Many comments addressed this issue with two arguments: (1) disputing the FDA's definition of what constitutes an implied disease claim; (2) contending that implied disease claims should be considered structure/function claims.

The FDA counters the first argument by stating that it has a long-standing history of interpreting implied disease claims as disease claims. In its proposed rule the FDA had requested comments regarding a particular type of implied disease claim for conditions that are not diseases themselves but rather are markers for or risk factors of disease. For example, the FDA considers "lowers cholesterol" to be an implied disease claim, whereas "helps maintain a healthy cholesterol level" is treated as a permissible structure/function claim. Most commenters agreed that consumers do not perceive a difference between these two claims. Dietary supplement manufacturers and some consumer groups concluded that both types of claims should therefore be permitted. In contrast, health professional groups, groups devoted to particular diseases, and other consumer groups contended that both types of claims should be prohibited.

The FDA opposes the second argument because it believes that consumers can readily link implied disease claims to the express disease, including serious and life-threatening diseases. The FDA feels this approach would lead to an undesirable situation in which: (1) consumers would be left to evaluate the validity of the implied disease claim; and (2) manufacturers of dietary supplements would have an unfair advantage over drug manufacturers, who are required to obtain premarket FDA approval of safety and efficacy for their products.

Labeling with citations to scientific references. In the FDA's final rule of January 6, 2000, it clarified the use of references to scientific literature. If the title cited implies that the product may have an effect on disease, then this labeling would be considered a disease claim. The FDA also indicated it would be considering "whether the cited article provides legitimate support for the express structure/function statement made . . . and whether citations are to bona fide research."[145]

The concurrence or permission of the FDA is not required for structure/function claims. However, the manufacturer must notify the FDA about the structure/function claim within the first thirty days of marketing the product. In the *Federal Register* of September 23, 1997, the FDA issued a final rule clarifying the requirements for notifications regarding structure/function claims. The FDA estimated that the burden on the manufacturer associated with this reporting process was 0.5 to 1 hour per notification.[146] This estimate was not disputed.[147] The structure/function claim must be truthful, not misleading, and based on scientific evidence contained in the manufacturer's substantiation file at the time the claim is made. Under DSHEA, manufacturers' substantiation files are not required to be accessible to the FDA.

DSHEA does not define how structure/function claims are to be substantiated. Because of the lack of patent protection and consequent lack of proprietary research on herbal products, structure/function claims tend to be defined in terms of the plant species contained in the product rather than the product's particular formulation. Substantiation is usually based on a history of use as well as research that is publicly available and often was conducted in other countries. The President's Commission on Dietary Supplement Labels suggested that structure/ function claims should be backed by scientifically valid evidence. The Commission indicated that structure/function claims based only on historical use should be "carefully qualified to prevent misleading consumers."[148] Without proposing that the rule making be reopened, the President's Commission on Dietary Supplement Labels suggested that manufacturers' substantiation files include the following items: a copy of the notification letter; the ingredients in the dietary supplement (including quantities and active principles if known); evidence to substantiate the statements of nutritional support; evidence to substantiate safety; Good Manufacturing Practices followed; and qualifications of the individuals who reviewed the evidence. The FDA agreed with this guidance but has no plans for rule revisions at this time.[149]

Health Claims

The Nutrition Labeling and Education Act of 1990 (NLEA)[150] established the procedures for approving health claims for foods. Unlike structure/function claims, health claims do require premarket

FDA approval. NLEA requires "significant scientific agreement" before a health claim is permitted on a food label. The Dietary Supplement Health and Education Act of 1994 left the standard for dietary supplement health claims up to the FDA's discretion, and the FDA applied the NLEA standard. In 1997, the President's Commission on Dietary Supplement Labels supported the FDA's position that the standard for health claims for both dietary supplements and foods should be "significant scientific agreement." However, the Commission clarified that "agreement" should not be interpreted to mean unanimous or near unanimous support and should include the opinions of experts outside the FDA. (The latter point was probably related to the fact that the FDA had lagged years behind the Centers for Disease Control and Prevention and Health and Human Services on accepting the scientific "agreement" about the link between folic acid deficiency and neural tube birth defects.) The health claim provisions of the Federal Food, Drug, and Cosmetic Act were further amended in the Food and Drug Administration Modernization Act of 1997, but most of the emphasis was on nonbotanical dietary supplements, such as vitamins and minerals.[123] Health claims that have been approved by the FDA in accordance with NLEA are limited to a short list based on extensive scientific data (on substances that would generally not be considered the active constituent in botanicals). Approved health claims for dietary supplements and conventional foods include: calcium and osteoporosis; folate and neural tube defects; soluble fiber from whole oats and coronary heart disease; and soluble fiber from psyllium husks and coronary heart disease. The President's Commission suggested that NLEA health claims be expanded to include appropriate health claims for herbal medicines.

Pearson v. Shalala. In this landmark case, on January 15, 1999, the United States Court of Appeals for the District of Columbia Circuit ruled against the FDA.[152] The suit was filed by Durk Pearson, Sandy Shaw, and the American Preventive Medical Association. Earlier, the FDA had decided to not authorize four health claims: (1) dietary fiber and cancer; (2) antioxidant vitamins and cancer; (3) omega-3 fatty acids and coronary heart disease; and (4) 0.8 mg folic acid in dietary supplement form is more effective in reducing the risk of neural tube defects than a lower amount in conventional food form. In their suit,

Pearson et al. challenged these decisions and the underlying health claim regulations.

The court ruled in favor of the plaintiffs on the grounds that "the first amendment does not permit FDA to reject health claims that the agency determines to be potentially misleading unless the agency also reasonably determines that no disclaimer would eliminate the potential deception."[153] The court required the FDA to: (a) reconsider their authorization decisions; and (b) clarify the standard for "significant scientific agreement." The FDA's first petition for a rehearing was denied on April 2, 1999. On December 1, 1999, the FDA issued its implementation strategy in the *Federal Register:* (1) update the scientific evidence on the four claims at issue in *Pearson v. Shalala;* (2) issue guidance clarifying the standard for "significant scientific agreement"; (3) hold a public meeting on the topic of health claim regulations; (4) conduct a rule making to reconsider the health claim regulations; and (5) conduct rule makings on the four Pearson health claims. These items were placed on the Center for Food Safety and Nutrition's Program Priorities List for 1999 and 2000.

By October 2000, the FDA had completed the first three steps,[154] including guidance for industry on the "significant scientific agreement" standard.[155] The FDA also revised its implementation strategy by establishing an interim enforcement strategy in which dietary supplement health claims would be considered at the FDA's discretion based on the following criteria:[156]

- a valid health claim petition has been filed;
- the scientific evidence in support of the claim outweighs the scientific evidence against the claim, the claim is appropriately qualified, and all statements in the claim are consistent with the weight of the scientific evidence;
- consumer health and safety are not threatened; and
- the claim meets the general requirements for health claims, except for the requirement that the evidence supporting the claim meet the significant scientific agreement standard and the requirement that the claim be made in accordance with an authorizing regulation.

On February 2, 2001, the U.S. District Court issued an opinion and order,[157] requiring the FDA to draft one or more "short, succinct, and accurate" disclaimers that could accompany the health claim for folic acid* on a label. The FDA complied but also filed a motion for reconsideration of the court's decision.

The health claims at issue in *Pearson v. Shalala* were not for botanicals. However, the fact that the court ruled against the FDA's interpretation of its own general health claim regulations may have implications for future cases involving botanical dietary supplements. The wait for such a case may not be long. On May 25, 1999, Dr. Julian Whitaker, Durk Pearson, Sandy Shaw, the American Preventive Medical Association, and Pure Encapsulation, Inc., submitted a petition to the FDA for the approval of saw palmetto (a botanical dietary supplement) for benign prostatic hypertrophy.[158]

Nutrient Content Labeling Requirements

The FDA's final rule on the labeling of the nutrient content of dietary supplements was issued in the *Federal Register* of September 23, 1997. All dietary supplement labels had to be in compliance with these requirements by March 23, 1999. The label requirements for dietary supplements were derived from the requirements for food labels with a few modifications. For example, under the new regulations dietary supplement labels must list total calories, calories from fat, total fat, saturated fat, cholesterol, sodium, total carbohydrate, dietary fiber, sugars, protein, vitamin A, vitamin C, calcium, and iron if the substance is present in the product above minimum threshold levels. (For foods these substances must be listed whether or not they are present in the product.) For botanical ingredients, the common name may be used if it is listed in the book *Herbs of Commerce*.[159] Otherwise, the Latin binomial (including author**) must be used. All ingredients must be listed, including those used solely for formulation. Extract solvents, ratios to starting material, plant part, and whether the starting material was fresh or dried must also be declared on the label. Certain aspects of the solvent declaration requirements were

---

*"0.8 mg folic acid in a dietary supplement is more effective in reducing the risk of neural tube defects than a lower amount in foods in common form."

**"Author" in botanical taxonomy refers to the person(s) who initially defined the species and, where applicable, revised the species definition since the original author's work. A Latin binomial that includes the author(s) is the soundest, most complete nomenclature for plant identification.

subsequently modified by the FDA in their final rule of June 5, 1998, in response to petitions from industry representatives.[160]

Alcohol Content

One final labeling issue arose concerning the alcohol content in some dietary supplement products. The Bureau of Alcohol, Tobacco, and Firearms (BATF) in the Department of Treasury regulates products that contain more than 0.5 percent alcohol and are fit for beverage use. The Food and Drug Administration (FDA) has authority over other products that contain alcohol. In response to reports of misuse of alcohol-containing ginseng extracts in New York, BATF has taken regulatory action to bring all ginseng products into compliance with federal labeling requirements with regard to declaring alcohol content.

Advertising

Advertising of herbal products in all media is governed by the Federal Trade Commission Act[161] and the Federal Trade Commission's criteria for support of food advertising claims.[162,163] Federal Trade Commission actions involving manufacturers of dietary supplement products have alleged violations in the form of deceptive acts or practices or unfair methods of competition in advertising through television, e-mail, and the Internet. In advertisements, representations (express or implied) about efficacy, performance, safety, or benefits must be substantiated by competent and reliable scientific evidence. An advertisement may not present an individual's testimonial as a typical user's experience without substantiation. Representations of dietary supplements in advertising must comply with the labeling regulations contained in the Nutrition Labeling and Education Act of 1990.

Exempt Publications

Under Section 5 of DSHEA, a publication or other reference may be used in connection with the sale of dietary supplements and is exempt from labeling restrictions if it meets the following requirements:

1. It is not false or misleading.
2. It does not promote a particular manufacturer or brand of a dietary supplement.
3. It is displayed or presented to convey a balanced view of the available scientific information on a dietary supplement.
4. If displayed in an establishment, it is displayed physically separate from the dietary supplements.
5. It does not have appended to it any additional information by sticker or any other method.

The Commission encouraged manufacturers to use third-party literature "to help consumers use dietary supplements appropriately."[164] The President's Commission noted the difficulties in applying this provision of DSHEA and suggested FDA proactively monitor this aspect. In the *Federal Register* of April 29, 1998, the FDA responded that they will be monitoring third-party literature but have no present plans for regulations.

Wholesale Distribution

Wholesale distribution of herbal products is governed by DSHEA. The confirmed adulteration of *Plantago lanceolata* L. with *Digitalis lanata* Ehrh. (see Chapter 9) highlights some of the problems that have arisen with respect to wholesale distribution of herbal products. In particular, that incident raised concern about the adequacy of existing systems with regard to proper identification and vouchering of botanicals, use of common names, record keeping, inaccurate certificates of analysis, economic adulteration, and postmarket surveillance.

Retail Sale

Until recently, herbal products were sold primarily in health food stores. The top-selling botanicals are now widely available in pharmacies, mass retail chain stores, and supermarkets. Several national brands of vitamins have launched herbal product lines. Many herbal products may be purchased in the offices of alternative health care practitioners. Specialty stores in some locations exclusively sell herbal products, raw plant material, and related books and magazines. Multilevel marketing is another retail channel for these products.

DSHEA governs dietary supplements that are involved in interstate commerce. Each state is responsible for locally produced and marketed products that do not enter interstate commerce. The retail sale of herbal products that contain more than 0.5 percent alcohol and are fit for use as a beverage may be controlled by the Bureau of Alcohol, Tobacco, and Firearms.

A wide variety of herbal products is available by mail order. Some of these products are grown and manufactured in the United States; others are imported. Several states expressed concern to the President's Commission on Dietary Supplement Labels about the uncontrolled information on herbal products that is available on the Internet.

Safety and Surveillance

Safety of dietary supplements, particularly botanicals, was a central issue during the congressional debates over DSHEA. Those on the regulatory side of the debate expressed concern that DSHEA hindered the FDA from protecting the public. Supplement proponents, however, claimed that the FDA had overstepped its regulatory bounds and misclassified herbs as "unsafe food additives." The congressional compromise articulated in DSHEA emphasized that the government should act quickly if a safety problem arises, but it should not impose unreasonable restrictions on access to safe supplement products.

Burden of Proof

Section 4 of the Dietary Supplement Health and Education Act of 1994 (DSHEA) established that the Food and Drug Administration (FDA) carries the burden of proving that a particular botanical product is unsafe. The President's Commission on Dietary Supplement Labels indicated that the "FDA and appropriate agencies in some States may need additional resources to develop the necessary evidence . . . to meet this important responsibility. . . ."[165] The FDA may remove a dietary supplement from the market if it can demonstrate that the product presents a significant or unreasonable risk of injury or illness when it is used as recommended on the label or, if it is not labeled, under conditions of ordinary use. An actual injury or illness need not have occurred before the FDA takes regulatory action. The

FDA may also oppose the marketing of a dietary supplement product if the label violates the regulations governing structure/function claims. The President's Commission on Dietary Supplement Labels strongly suggested to manufacturers that they include appropriate warnings in product information. The FDA Foods Advisory Committee, together with industry, is developing guidance on this matter. Examples illustrating some of the nuances of the safety issues in practice are described in more detail in Chapter 9.

Presidential Commission's Policy Guidance on Safety

The Commission's report underscored the safety of botanicals saying "there are relatively few reports in the scientific literature that indicate potential or actual toxicity following the use of these products. When such reports are found, they often are single-case reports involving an allergenic reaction or toxicity due to improper labeling, or adulteration, or an idiosyncratic reaction. . . ."[166] They made no safety recommendations (for proposed rule) but offered the following Policy Guidance: (1) the supplement industry must accept the responsibility of assuring that supplements are and will continue to be safe; (2) the FDA, industry, scientists, and consumer groups should cooperate in the development of postmarket surveillance systems so that adverse reactions can be reported and corrected quickly; (3) manufacturers should include appropriate warnings on labels; (4) the FDA should quickly address known safety issues (such as products containing ephedrine alkaloids); and (5) federal and state agencies may need additional resources for investigations in the context of their overall health priorities.

Postmarket Surveillance

Several large-scale, passive surveillance systems monitor adverse reactions to all foods, including dietary supplements. Reporting to any of these systems is voluntary and carries no legal obligations. Manufacturers are not required to report adverse events. Consumer reports of adverse events associated with herbal products are currently accepted by the Poison Control Centers and the FDA.

- The U.S. Pharmacopoeia maintains a Practitioners' Reporting Network for clinicians.
- The Association of Poison Control Centers monitors all adverse reactions reported to the national network of Poison Control Centers.
- The Food and Drug Administration (FDA) enters all reports of adverse events related to dietary supplements that they receive into the Center for Food Safety and Applied Nutrition's (CFSAN) Special Nutritionals Adverse Event Monitoring System for further evaluation and monitoring.
- The FDA uses its MedWatch system to track serious adverse events that are associated with dietary supplements (and other FDA-regulated products).
- The FDA also receives passive surveillance data on adverse events associated with foods and dietary supplements through the Drug Quality Reporting System and the Office of Regulatory Affairs Consumer Complaint System.

In April 2001, the Office of the Inspector General in the U.S. Department of Health and Human Services issued its assessment of the FDA's adverse event reporting system for dietary supplements.[167] The report concluded that the existing system "cannot serve as an adequate safety valve."[168] Among the findings based on the analysis of FDA data on adverse event reports from 1994 through 1999 were the following: [169]

- Adverse event reports received by the FDA from health professionals: 20 percent
- Adverse event reports received by the FDA from manufacturers: fewer than 10
- Reported products for which ingredients could not be determined: 32 percent
- Reported products for which labels could not be obtained: 77 percent
- Reported products for which samples had been requested but not received: 69 percent
- Reported products for which the manufacturer could not be determined: 32 percent

- Manufacturers for which the city and state could not be found: 71 percent
- Reports that were flagged as needing follow-up but could not be pursued because of insufficient information about the individual involved: 27 percent

The President's Commission on Dietary Supplement Labels recommended that the FDA, industry, scientists, and consumer groups cooperate in the establishment of a postmarket surveillance system specifically for dietary supplements. In the *Federal Register* of April 29, 1998, the FDA stated that it will initiate a process to further such cooperation. An internal working group of the FDA's Foods Advisory Committee (comprised of outside experts) has been asked to address the question of postmarket surveillance.

Strategic Plans of the FDA and the Office of Dietary Supplements (ODS)

In June 1998, the FDA and CFSAN held a stakeholders meeting where three basic themes were identified:

(1) the need to maintain a credible FDA program, including compliance, enforcement, and consumer outreach activities that will help ensure consumer confidence in FDA regulated products; (2) the need to maintain a solid, science based program staffed with highly qualified scientists; and (3) the recognition that FDA's assistance to consumers and the regulated industry is important.[170]

The 1999 Program Priorities for CFSAN called for

the development of an overall dietary supplement strategy in conjunction with other agency units and stakeholders [that] . . . should address all elements of the dietary supplement program including: (1) Boundaries between dietary supplement and conventional foods, between dietary supplements and drugs, and between dietary supplements and cosmetic products; (2) claims; (3) good manufacturing practices; (4) adverse event reporting; (5) laboratory capability; (6) research needs; (7) enforcement; and

(8) resource needs. . . . FDA has identified four criteria for priority ranking the tasks encompassed in the strategy. These criteria are: (1) enhancement of consumer safety, (2) development of health-related product labeling regulation, (3) improvement in efficiency of operation, and (4) closure on unresolved regulatory issues.[171]

Toward these ends, FDA has held two public meetings, one in Washington, DC, on June 8, 1999, and the other in Oakland, California, on July 20, 1999. The meeting attendees were requested to address the following questions:

1. In addition to ensuring consumer access to safe dietary supplements that are truthfully and not misleadingly labeled, are there other objectives that an overall dietary supplement strategy should include? 2. Are the criteria for prioritizing the tasks within the supplement strategy appropriate? Which specific tasks should FDA undertake first? 3. What factors should FDA consider in determining how best to implement a task (i.e., use of regulations, guidance, etc.)? 4. What tasks should be included under the various dietary supplement program elements in the CFSAN 1999 Program Priorities documents? 5. Are there current safety, labeling, or other marketplace issues that FDA should address quickly through enforcement actions to ensure, for example, that consumers have confidence that the products on the market are safe and truthfully and not misleadingly labeled? 6. Toward what type or area of research on dietary supplements should FDA allocate its research resources? 7. Given FDA's limited resources, what mechanisms are available, or should be developed, to leverage FDA's resources to meet effectively the objective of the strategy?[172]

The FDA's Ten-Year Dietary Supplement Strategy

In January 2000, the FDA and the Center for Food Safety and Applied Nutrition issued their ten-year plan for dietary supplements.[138] The program goal is as follows: "By the year 2010, [have] a science-based regulatory program that fully implements the Dietary Supplement Health and Education Act of 1994, thereby providing consumers with a high level of confidence in the safety, composition, and labeling of dietary supplement products."[174] The plan includes an ambitious list of loosely defined tasks needed to complete the unfinished business of implementing DSHEA. The strategy is divided among the general headings of safety, labeling, boundaries, enforcement activities, science-base, and outreach. Only the boundaries section specifically mentions botanicals: "Develop a regulatory framework for botanicals used in traditional/alternative medicine (including how they relate to over-the-counter drugs)."[175]

ODS Status Report and Strategic Plan

The first director of the ODS issued a status report for the years 1995-1998 and a strategic plan for the next three to five years. In the strategic plan she emphasized that more research on botanicals ("nonnutrient dietary supplements") is badly needed. Given the high cost of clinical trials and the much lower cost of epidemiological studies, she suggested "epidemiological studies of supplement exposures and specific health outcomes" would be a good place to start. The results could then guide subsequent clinical trials. She also stressed that the government cannot be the sole source of research funding for dietary supplements. Collaboration among academia, industry, and various government agencies is needed. On October 25, 1999, the second director of the ODS was appointed.

Nutraceutical Research and Education Act

Representative Frank Pallone (D-New Jersey) introduced the Nutraceutical Research and Education Act (NREA) in the House on October 1, 1999. The bill intended to amend the FDC Act "to promote clinical research and development on dietary supplements and foods for their health benefits; to establish a new legal classification for dietary supplements and food with health benefits, and for other purposes."[176] The bill proposed a legal definition for nutraceuticals that references the Orphan Drug Act,[177] a definition of "health benefit," a simplified process for approving health benefits of nutraceuticals, a ten-year period of exclusive marketing protection, and the establishment of an Advisory Council on Nutraceuticals. The scientific evidence required to support a "health benefit" of a nutraceutical product would be determined by the advisory council on a case-by-case basis. It would include at least one clinical trial of "a sufficient size to prove the benefits and may have as its endpoints either surrogate markers or clinical endpoints to support the claim. The application may also include epidemiological or preclinical studies. . . ."[178]

Although NREA was not reintroduced in the 107th Congress, its concepts suggest that there is an ongoing concern among some in Washington about DSHEA's limitations.

Chapter 3

Canada

Canada is well along in the process of overhauling its regulation of "natural health products" (NHPs), which include botanicals.[1,2] These changes were initiated in response to several pressures, including consumer demand, efforts at international harmonization, and problems associated with Canada's close proximity to the U.S market, where these products are regulated as dietary supplements (foods). A summary of Canada's progress follows.

In May 1997, Health Canada established the Advisory Panel on Natural Health Products.* That same year, the Minister of Health requested that the House of Commons Standing Committee on Health thoroughly review Canadian regulation of NHPs. By the end of 1997, the Therapeutic Products Programme (TPP), which regulates pharmaceutical drugs, had submitted a background report to the Committee. The Advisory Panel on Natural Health Products issued its findings in May 1998, and the Standing Committee on Health issued its final report on this topic in November 1998.[3] The Committee set out the following principles as guidelines for its position.

- *Nature of NHPs:* NHPs are different in nature from and must not be treated strictly as either food or pharmaceutical products.
- *Safety:* Safety of NHPs is of primary concern.
- *Quality:* The NHP industry must meet clearly defined and established standards of quality.
- *Access:* NHP regulations must not unduly restrict access by consumers.
- *Informed Choice:* NHP consumers must be provided with pertinent information about the products they purchase.

---

*The Advisory Panel on Natural Health Products was initially named the Advisory Panel on Herbal Remedies.

- *Cost:* NHP regulations must not place inappropriate cost on industry, consumers, and government.
- *Decision Making:* Decision-making power must be given to a regulatory body with expertise and experience with NHPs.
- *Availability of Appeal:* An open and transparent process of appeal must be available to NHP stakeholders.
- *Transparency:* Information regarding decisions and the regulatory system must be readily available to NHP stakeholders.
- *Cultural Diversity:* NHP regulations must respect diverse cultural traditions.[4]

In April 1999, the Minister of Health accepted all fifty-three of the Standing Committee's recommendations (see Appendix B for a complete list of the Committee's recommendations). By May 1999, the Ministry of Health had established a Transition Team to oversee the creation of an Office of Natural Health Products (ONHP), develop a regulatory framework for natural health products, and select an executive director. Fourteen of the team's seventeen members came from the private sector.

The Transition Team took a wellness rather than a disease approach to the model, and established the following mission statement for the ONHP in August 1999:

> The Mission of the Office of Natural Health Products is to ensure that Canadians have ready access to natural health products that are safe, effective, and of high quality while respecting freedom of choice and philosophical and cultural diversity.[5]

The federal government allotted $10 million to the ONHP for a three-year period.

In January 2000, Health Canada announced the new Executive Director of the Office of Natural Health Products, a doctor of naturopathic medicine with a master's degree in business administration. Reporting to the executive director are four areas: Policy and Regulatory Affairs; Research and Program Development; Outreach and Communications; and Product Regulation. An Expert Advisory Committee (EAC) representing a range of disciplines* supports all four areas. The ONHP was later renamed the Natural Health Products Directorate. It is now structured alongside but separate from the Food Directorate and the Therapeutic Products Directorate. All three of these Directorates report to the Health Products and Food Branch of Health Canada.

The Transition Team concluded their work in March 2000, issuing a final report[6] with recommendations on mission, vision, organizational structure, a regulatory framework, modifications to existing regulations, research, and communications as well as several position statements. Their recommendations incorporated comments from a wide range of stakeholders. Before disbanding, they suggested that an Interim Management Policy for regulating natural health products be implemented immediately, while the permanent rules are being developed.

In December 2001, Health Minister Allan Rock announced the new regulations, labeling requirements, the transfer of approximately 25,000 natural health products to the jurisdiction of the Natural Health Products Directorate (with a two-year transition period), and $800,000** per year in research funding starting in 2002-2003 ($400,000 in partnership with the Canadian Institutes of Health Research and $400,000 for Health Canada to fund specific research initiatives).[7] The proposed regulations were created as a new set of regulations under the Food and Drugs Act. They were published in the *Canada Gazette,* Part I, on December 22, 2001. A ninety-day comment period followed. Once the final regulations are published in the *Canada Gazette,* Part II, transition provisions will go into effect immediately and full compliance will be required within two years.

Similar to the United States, Canada has chosen to create a legal category that is separate from both food and drugs. Yet in distinct contrast to the United States, Canada elected to establish a regulatory system that requires premarket approval for these products. Consumer demand is a major driver in the Canadian market for natural health products, as it is in the United States. A poll conducted in

---

*Disciplines sought for the Expert Advisory Panel include: medicine, naturopathy, pharmacy, herbalists, manufacturing/importers, traditional Chinese medicine, toxicology, pharmacognosy, homeopathy, phytochemistry, consumer representation, epidemiology, biochemistry, orthomolecular nutrition, growers, sports medicine, and Ayurveda.

**Dollar amounts represent Canadian currency.

August 1997 found that 67 percent of Canadians were in favor of federal regulation of the quality and safety of natural health products.[8] A national survey in 1997 indicated 56 percent of Canadians reported they had taken at least one natural health product in the previous six months; this included 20 percent who had taken an herbal remedy or tea.[9] The Canadian market for natural health products is estimated to exceed $1.5 billion, of which 30 percent is attributed to botanicals.[10] Still, consumer representatives reported to the Standing Committee on Health that they felt their government was denying them access to beneficial products.

Each section of the following review of the Canadian regulations presents the existing regulations first, then describes the proposed regulations published in the *Canada Gazette* on December 22, 2001.

LEGAL CLASSIFICATION

Existing Regulations

In Canada, herbal medicinal products are not yet legally defined. They have been regulated for general sale as either a food or a drug under the Food and Drugs Act of 1952. The distinction between food and drug is primarily based on whether a therapeutic claim is made. With a therapeutic claim, the product is considered a drug. Without a claim, it is regulated as a food. Examples of botanicals that are considered foods include herbal teas and candies.

Herbal products that are considered drugs generally have pharmacological properties that could lead to side effects, and they tend to be taken as remedies rather than as a part of the diet. Most botanical OTC drugs are traditional; only one has been authorized for new uses.* Although none have been approved, in principle herbal substances may be mixed with vitamins or minerals if the indications, dosage, and directions are justified. (Vitamins and minerals are currently regulated as drugs.)

---

*As of 1998, Ginsana was the only botanical approved as a nontraditional OTC drug. Its active ingredient is standardized ginsennosides. The authorized indication is to assist with recuperation from long periods of inactivity following an illness and to help hand/eye coordination when inhibited in the elderly.

Traditional herbal medicines (THMs) are currently regulated as drugs under a specific set of guidelines issued in 1990 and 1995.[11,12] THMs are over-the-counter finished drug products that are generally used for self-medication of self-limiting conditions. Their active ingredients are botanicals with traditional uses that are well-documented in herbal references but not necessarily in the scientific literature. The combination of active principles in a THM may be questioned if it is likely to have multiple or contradictory effects. The nonactive ingredients in THMs may be chemically defined or botanical. The label on THM products must state "traditional herbal medicine used for . . ." THMs that do not comply with the guidelines are treated as "new drugs," which are regulated as pharmaceuticals are under Division 8 of the Food and Drug Regulations.

Homeopathic drugs are regulated under distinct guidelines published in 1990.[13] They must be labeled as homeopathic preparations that are "to be used as directed by a physician" or "by a homeopathic practitioner." Combining botanicals and homeopathic ingredients is prohibited. If a homeopathic drug does not comply with the guidelines, then it falls under Division 8 of the Food and Drug Regulations.

Proposed Natural Health Product Regulations

In the new proposed regulations,[14] natural health products (NHPs) are defined by their intended use and by their ingredient(s). Products are considered NHPs when marketed for use in:

- the diagnosis, treatment, mitigation, or prevention of a disease, disorder, or abnormal physical state or its symptoms in humans;
- restoring or correcting organic functions in humans; or
- maintaining or promoting health or otherwise modifying organic functions in humans.

Homeopathic preparations and traditional medicines are classified as NHPs. However, the NHP definition and regulations do not apply to health care practitioners (e.g., pharmacists, aboriginal healers, traditional Chinese medicine practitioners, herbalists, naturopathic doctors) who compound products for specific patients. The inclusion list specifies the medicinal ingredients that are permitted in NHPs, and the exclusion list stipulates prohibited ingredients.

Inclusion List for Natural Health Products

    a. a plant or plant material, alga, fungus, or non-human animal material
    b. an extract or isolate of a), the primary molecular structure of which is the same as that which it had prior to its extraction or isolation
    c. a vitamin (a term which is defined in the regulations), or any of its salts or derivatives
    d. an amino acid or any of its salts
    e. an essential fatty acid
    f. a synthetic duplicate of b) to e)
    g. a mineral
    h. a probiotic

New drug substances from the inclusion list that have been chemically altered after extraction from a natural source are not considered NHPs, unless they are conjugates or salts. Substances from the inclusion list that have narrow margins of safe dosages are also excluded from the definition of NHPs.

Exclusion List for Natural Health Products

- an antibiotic
- a substance intended for injection
- a substance regulated under the *Tobacco Act*
- a substance described in Schedule C (radiopharmaceuticals)
- a substance described in Schedule D (biologics)

Botanicals sold in bulk form are classified as NHPs—not foods. The Food Directorate and Natural Health Product Directorate will be issuing a list of herbs that have no recognized food purpose and are therefore considered to be NHPs—not foods. Products in a food medium are considered to be foods—rather than NHPs—if they are primarily consumed to provide nourishment, nutrition or hydration, or to satisfy hunger, thirst, or a desire for taste, texture, or flavor.

PROOF OF SAFETY AND EFFICACY

Existing Regulations

Herbal products that are sold as foods do not need premarket approval. However, a list of approximately sixteen herbs and botanical preparations is considered unacceptable for use as foods or ingredients in foods.[15] These assessments were mainly based on toxicological and epidemiological evidence.

All drugs offered for general sale, including herbal medicinal products with therapeutic claims, are regulated under the Food and Drugs Act and the Food and Drug Regulations. After receiving premarket approval of quality, safety, efficacy, labeling, and package inserts and paying a fee, drugs are assigned a Drug Identification Number (DIN). These laws do not cover products that are compounded or dispensed for a particular individual after consultation with a practitioner. This exemption also applies to aboriginal healers who administer botanicals extemporaneously to individuals in their communities. However, restricted substances are not permitted to be used in these preparations.

Nontraditional herbal medicinal products are held to the same standards as pharmaceutical drugs. They must file New Drug Submissions under Division 8 of the Food and Drug Regulations. The type of evidence required depends on the availability of data. For well-known substances with a particular nonprescription indication, the manufacturer need only reference a published monograph standard. If such a standard does not exist, then published data, including references to traditional uses, may be provided instead. When the ingredient is well known but the indication is new, then clinical data and sometimes new safety data are required. If the substance is new, a full application must be submitted, including clinical, safety, and formulation data. Very few botanicals have the necessary data required to enter the market through this route.

No product that combines botanical ingredients with vitamins or minerals has been approved. However, in principle, manufacturers of such products must justify the combination's use, dosage, and directions. For instance, vitamins or minerals would not be acceptable in combination with laxative botanicals for two reasons: first, the laxative effect would reduce absorption of the micronutrients; second, laxatives should not be used daily.

Traditional herbal medicines (THMs) fall under separate guidelines for safety and efficacy,[16] although they also receive DINs. First, there can be no recent evidence of toxicity. Second, applications for THMs may not cite scientific studies. Only references to traditional uses and dosages are accepted. If scientific citations are used, then the application is treated as a New Drug Submission, as a pharmaceutical would be. References must be provided to substantiate the safety and indications claimed. For each botanical ingredient, photocopies of two references to traditional use must be provided. Also, a photocopy of the herbal monograph must be submitted. The monograph has to state the pharmacological activity, therapeutic use, part of the plant used, daily and single dose for that part of the plant, and dosage form. For combination products, the guidelines for THMs do not allow the active ingredients to have multiple effects (e.g., laxative and diuretic) or contradictory effects (e.g., laxatives and astringents).[13] Each botanical ingredient is evaluated individually. Ingredients that have similar effects are considered to have additive effects in the combination. Finally, the product must be suitable for use in self-medication with a purpose that consumers can readily understand.

Proposed Natural Health Product Regulations

The proposed regulations require that all natural health products have product licenses prior to marketing. Licensing would involve compliance with standards for safety and claims (as well as quality, labeling, and postmarket surveillance, which are discussed later in this chapter). Once the final regulations are published, companies would be required to notify the Natural Health Product Directorate of any NHPs currently being sold. The company could then continue to market the NHP (unless health or safety concerns arose) until it received its product license. All products would have to be licensed within two years.

Standards of Evidence

The Standing Committee on Health proposed a premarket assessment system for natural health products that is more rigorous than food evaluations but less stringent than the drug approval process. The Transition Team further developed this notion and indicated that standards of evidence should be: "a function of the quality of the individual studies, as well as the quantity, quality, consistency and strength of the overall data available and their relevance to the claim . . . sufficiently rigorous to protect public health interest and enhance consumer confidence . . . [and] flexible to allow industry to develop useful products at a reasonable cost and to accommodate changing scientific developments."[18] The Transition Team specifically recommended that:

- The evidence to support the safety and claim of a product must not be limited to double-blind clinical trials, but may also include other types of evidence, such as generally accepted and traditional references, published monographs, expert opinion reports, other types of clinical trials and other clinical or scientific evidence;
- the ONHP, with the assistance of the EAC, should establish a list of acceptable references, develop the criteria for ONHP-approved monographs and develop criteria for linking levels of evidence to health claim validity; and,
- claim approval by the ONHP, on the basis of scientific evidence, should be allowed to be applied to other products, with supportive scientific evidence of at least an equal level of claim assessment.[19]

The proposed NHP regulations include safety standards, which are described in the next section. The Natural Health Product Directorate has not yet released standards of evidence for claims.

Minimum Safety Standard

The Standing Committee recognized that the vast majority of botanicals are considered to be safe. For these products, the expense of toxicological or clinical studies would be unnecessary. Instead, they recommended focusing resources on assessing products that present the greatest risk. The Committee recommended that products be categorized on the basis of risk. Products in the lower risk category would be subject to less rigorous premarket and postmarket standards. Higher risk products would require thorough premarket data packages and active, rigorous postmarket surveillance.

Under the new regulations, products that do not meet minimum safety standards would not be considered NHPs and would be regulated as drugs by the Therapeutic Products Programme. More specifically, a product would not be an NHP if the difference between its recommended dose and its toxic dose is too small. This standard is defined in the proposed regulations as the margin between:

- the lowest dose at which it produces toxicity in humans; and
- the highest dose at which it does not produce toxicity in humans.[20]

Information forming the basis for such a determination may be drawn from:

- its recorded history of use in humans;
- its clinical experience data;
- its adverse reaction reports; and
- its toxicological effects in any animal species tested.[21]

Permissible Claims

The Standing Committee recognized three types of health claims for natural health products, and these are reflected in the definition of NHPs in the new regulations.

- *Structure/function claims* are for products that promote health by improving the structure or physiological function of the human body. Example: "Calcium builds strong bones."
- *Risk reduction claims* are for products that promote health either by a reducing a recognized risk factor or by increasing the body's resistance to disease. Example: "Garlic decreases the risk of cardiovascular diseases."
- *Therapeutic or treatment claims* are for products that cure a disease or alleviate the symptoms of a disease. Example: "St. John's wort is useful in the treatment of mild to moderate depression."

Products may also be sold without claims, provided they meet safety and quality standards.

Efficacy Standards in Monographs

The Standing Committee and the Transition Team sought an approach that would allow resources to be focused primarily on new products and nonstandard claims. For assessment of lower risk products, the Standing Committee recommended relying on the monographs available in Canada or other countries. Products that complied with these monographs would need no further evidence of efficacy, and the regulating authority would have a shorter time than usual (e.g., thirty days) to finalize the approval. The Committee further suggested that standardized Canadian monographs be developed and eventually be compiled into a Canadian pharmacopoeia or compendium. Data from Canada or other countries would be permitted. The Committee saw no reason to duplicate the effort that had already gone into monographs in other countries, provided the foreign data were reviewed by knowledgeable Canadians.

The proposed NHP regulations include a sixty-day disposition clause or performance standard, which would require the Directorate to process within sixty days those applications that reference monographs. The monographs are based on publicly available data and may cover products that contain a single or multiple medicinal ingredients.

Efficacy Standards in the Absence of Monographs

In the absence of a monograph, the Standing Committee and the Transition Team recommended that the level of evidence required should correlate with the degree of risk presented by the product and the type of claim. Higher risk products or more serious claims would require more rigorous data. The Transition Team proposed that evaluators of NHPs weigh risk within the context of claim and usage and consider whether:

- individualized instructions and/or practitioner supervision or monitoring is required to ensure safety or effectiveness;

- there is a narrow margin of safety between therapeutic dose and toxic dose;
- there is significant potential for undesirable or severe side effects at normal therapeutic dosage levels;
- known experimental data has shown that the product induces toxicity in animals, but the product has not been in clinical use long enough to establish the pattern of long-term toxic effects in humans;
- safe use is known to possibly mask other serious ailment(s) or their development;
- statistically significant potential for addiction, abuse, severe dependency or other harmful effects has been demonstrated;
- they possess a low level of safety relative to expected benefits; and,
- whether they have a therapeutic effect based on recently established pharmacological concepts, the consequence of which has not yet been fully established.[22]

The NHP Directorate will be issuing clarification of the necessary standards for all types of NHP claims. The proposed NHP regulations note that the efficacy of botanicals is influenced by numerous factors (e.g., growing conditions of the plant, the part of the plant, extraction methods, dosage form) and therefore claims made for one extract cannot be transferred to another extract without specific efficacy data.[23] The proposed NHP regulations also include clinical trial requirements and good clinical practice standards.[24]

MANUFACTURING STANDARDS

Existing Regulations

All foods, including herbal products without therapeutic claims, must follow the voluntary food guidelines for good manufacturing practices. Herbal medicinal products that are marketed as drugs must comply with the same good manufacturing practices as all drugs.[25] Canada has developed additional guidelines[26] that are specific to herbal medicinal products based on the World Health Organization (WHO) guidelines.[27]

Drug manufacturers, importers, fabricators, packagers, distributors, and testers are all required to maintain an establishment license. However, the producers of natural health products have been exempt from this licensing requirement during the regulatory overhaul. GMP requirements still apply.

Proposed Natural Health Product Regulations

The Standing Committee on Health made several recommendations related to manufacturing standards. First, it suggested that Health Canada and industry work together to create GMP guidelines that reflect the specific needs for natural health products in general and botanicals in particular. Second, it proposed that establishment licenses be required for all manufacturers, packagers, importers, and distributors of natural health products sold in Canada, regardless of whether the business operates in Canada or elsewhere. Third, it recommended that inspectors be specifically trained in natural health products and then conduct regular inspections.

The proposed NHP regulations require a site license for any building in which "an NHP is imported, distributed, manufactured, packaged, labeled, or stored prior to sale."[28] Growers and wholesalers would be exempt. After the final regulations are published, companies that have existing sites will be required to immediately notify the NHP Directorate about their sites and then obtain a site license within two years. New sites would require a license before going into operation. The site licensing system is designed to cover the entire supply chain, to assure quality, to assist with product recalls as needed, to treat foreign and Canadian players similarly, and to set resource requirements in accordance with the fact that NHPs tend to present a lower risk than pharmaceuticals. Among other requirements, site licensing involves compliance with good manufacturing practices (GMPs).

The proposed NHP regulations define GMPs in terms of outcomes. Subsequently, on April 17, 2002, the NHP Directorate issued draft guidance on GMPs[29] that spells out each requirement more specifically. Comments on the draft are being accepted through August 18, 2002. The NHP Directorate also plans to establish GMP equivalencies with other countries by developing MOUs (memoranda of understanding) with foreign site inspection authorities and MRAs (mutual recognition agreements) with foreign regulatory agencies.

LABELING, ADVERTISING, DISTRIBUTION, AND RETAIL SALE

Labeling

Existing Regulations

For herbal products marketed as foods, no therapeutic claims are permitted on the label or promotional material. Labels on traditional herbal medicine products must include the phrase "traditional herbal medicine used for . . . .". Otherwise, the usual labeling guidelines for drugs also apply to herbal medicinal products. Labeling and package inserts, including therapeutic claims, must be authorized as part of the DIN approval process. In practice, however, unapproved claims do appear on labels, displays, and product brochures, especially on botanical foods. (Technically such claims would render these products drugs, but since they have not undergone premarket approval they are being sold illegally as foods.)

Proposed Natural Health Product Regulations

The Standing Committee on Health recommended that labels be required to clearly state the type of supporting evidence for the health claim made (e.g., traditional use, clinical use, scientific studies, etc.). The Committee felt this requirement would serve several purposes. First, it would allow consumers to make more informed choices about products. Second, it would give the industry an incentive to conduct research on their products. Third, it would level the playing field and promote fair competition among pharmaceuticals and natural health products.

The Committee found that current restrictions on the labeling of natural health products made it more difficult for consumers to make informed choices. It considered more complete labeling and package insert information to be a foundation for its risk management approach to regulating natural health products.

The proposed NHP regulations address these concerns by establishing, as a condition of licensure, labeling requirements that "will assist consumers in selecting products that meet their particular needs and expectations, and in understanding the merits and limitations of the products they choose."[30] Specifically, labels would be required to include the following information (items marked with an asterisk (*) are required on small packages):

- the brand name;*
- the product number (issued with the product license, preceded by the designation NHP or PSN);*
- the dosage form;
- if the NHP is sterile, the notations "sterile" and "stérile";*
- if the NHP is one which is available for sale on prescription, the symbol "Pr";*
- the net amount of the NHP in terms of weight, measure, or number;*
- the name and address of the product license holder;
- if the NHP is imported, the name and address of the importer (and the product license holder);
- the proper name and, if any, the common name of each medicinal ingredient;*
- the strength or potency of the medicinal ingredients (by proper name);
- a qualitative list of all nonmedicinal ingredients;
- the recommended use or purpose (in English and French);*
- the recommended route of administration (in English and French);
- the recommended dose and, if any, the duration of use (in English and French);*
- the risk information relating to the NHP, including any cautions, warnings, contra-indications, or known adverse reactions associated with the use of that NHP (in English and French);
- the recommended storage conditions, if any;
- the lot number;*
- the expiration date;*
- a description of the source material from which the medicinal ingredients are derived or obtained (for example, root of plant).[31]

Advertising

Existing Regulations

Advertising of drugs to the general public is permitted, except for products intended to treat the diseases on a specific list ("Schedule A") that are considered to require the involvement of a medical professional. Under the Food and Drugs Act, representation of food and drugs may not be false, misleading, or deceptive. For herbal medicinal products, unapproved claims are prohibited in advertising just as they are in labeling. Advertising for botanical drugs requires preclearance by a third party, but the process is voluntary. Guidelines for the advertising of botanical foods exist but are voluntary.

Proposed NHP Regulations

The proposed regulations do not address advertising. However, the Standing Committee on Health called for a study of Schedule A to see whether it was still serving a purpose. The Committee indicated that other aspects of its recommendations may have eliminated the need for Schedule A to protect the public from natural health products intended to treat serious conditions. The Transition Team subsequently proposed that Schedule A be revoked, noting that it constrained disease prevention efforts.[32] The proposed NHP regulations did not include this change, but discussions about how best to modify Schedule A are ongoing.

Distribution and Retail Sale

Existing Regulations

Currently there are no restrictions on where herbal medicinal products may be sold. These types of restrictions would be instated at the provincial level. Natural health products are bought in health food stores, supplement and nutrition stores, practitioners' offices, pharmacies, drugstores, grocery stores, and through network marketing, via mail order, and over the Internet. The Food and Drugs Act has a provision that permits an individual to import drug products for personal use. Importation and distribution of unapproved products have been regulatory concerns in Canada. The problem arises when products that are bought from other countries (especially the United States) for personal use do not meet Canadian standards for claims, quality, safety, and efficacy.

Proposed NHP Regulations

The Standing Committee on Health concluded that the problems with imported products would probably be alleviated when more natural health products were approved for the Canadian market. However, after their regulatory revisions are implemented, they recommended that the issue of importation for personal use be revisited.

The Committee envisioned a system in which products designated as higher risk would be controlled either by additional labeling stipulations and/or by requiring a product to be purchased from a practitioner. The labels describe the risks and recommend that consumers consult a qualified practitioner prior to using the product. The highest-risk products would be available only through a practitioner. However, this proposal would be problematic to implement in Canada because few practitioners that administer natural health products are regulated and this type of authority is under the jurisdiction of the provinces.

The proposed NHP regulations are not intended to govern the retail sale of NHPs.

POSTMARKET SAFETY AND SURVEILLANCE

Existing Regulations

The Canadian Food Inspection Agency considers botanicals that are sold as foods to represent a very small risk relative to the entire food system. Monitoring these products is therefore considered a low priority.

The current postmarket surveillance system was designed to monitor prescription drugs, so medical professionals are actively involved in reporting. In principle, an adverse reaction to any drug can be reported. However, in practice, patients usually do not inform their physicians about their use of botanicals and few reports on herbal medicines have been submitted.

Canada has withdrawn several herbal medicines, such as comfrey, in response to adverse event reports in other countries. Ephedra has been recalled on a voluntary basis. Earlier restrictions had been placed on its dosage and indications, and the label had to include a cautionary statement.

Proposed Natural Health Product Regulations

As mentioned previously, the Standing Committee on Health recommended categorizing botanicals on the basis of risk. Lower risk products would be monitored with adverse event reports. Products presenting higher risk would be subject to more frequent and more rigorous surveillance. Manufacturers would be required to maintain and analyze postmarket data on their products, including data on interactions with other natural health products, pharmaceuticals, and foods. The Committee also proposed establishing a user-friendly adverse event hotline for practitioners and the general public.

The proposed NHP regulations would define three types of adverse events:

1. "adverse reaction" means a noxious and unintended response to a natural health product that occurs at any dose used or tested for the diagnosis, treatment, or prevention of a disease or for modifying an organic function.
2. "serious adverse reaction" means a noxious and unintended response to a natural health product that occurs at any dose and that requires inpatient hospitalization or a prolongation of existing hospitalization, that causes congenital malformation, that results in persistent or significant disability or incapacity, that is life threatening, or that results in death.
3. "serious unexpected adverse reaction" means a serious adverse reaction that is not identified in nature, severity, or frequency in the risk information set out on the label of the natural health product.[33]

For the latter two types, a case report would have to be submitted within fifteen days of becoming aware of the event. Companies would be required to compile annual reports of adverse reactions at the labeled dose and to submit these reports to the Minister of Health upon request.[34] The holder of the product license would be responsible for observing any patterns in adverse reactions.

Chapter 4

Germany

LEGAL CLASSIFICATION

In Germany, the Second Medicines Law of 1976 governs all medicinal products, including herbal medicinal products.[1] Herbal medicinal products contain only plant material in crude or processed form. However, single chemical constituents isolated from plants (e.g., menthol) are not considered herbal medicinal products. All herbal medicinal products have a therapeutic or prophylactic claim.

Foods are generally not treated as medicines.[2] Products are defined as medicines or foods based on their intended use. The primary criteria for this distinction include common opinion, composition, recommended dose, and therapeutic or prophylactic claims. The secondary criteria are labeling, place of sale, and price. A product such as peppermint tea may be sold as an herbal medicinal product with therapeutic or prophylactic claims, or as a beverage (i.e., food).

Products may not combine homeopathic and herbal ingredients. Mixtures of herbal medicinal ingredients with food or cosmetics are also prohibited. However, there are some combination products (e.g., botanicals mixed with homeopathics, vitamins, or minerals) that have been on the market for many years and are regulated as drugs. These products may have difficulty with registration renewals in the future because they are combinations of substances in different legal categories.

PROOF OF SAFETY AND EFFICACY

All medicinal products, including herbal medicinal products, require premarket approval of quality, safety, and efficacy in line with

European and German legislation.[3] The German treatment of herbal medicinal products is somewhat analogous to the American OTC process in that there is one procedure for "old" products that were already on the market when the legislation was passed and another protocol for "new" products. This section begins with a brief regulatory history, then describes the situation for old products, followed by new products.

Regulatory History

Medicines Law of 1976 (Instituted in 1978)

This legislation defined herbal medicines as medicinal products and required them to be registered with the federal health authority. Products that were already marketed prior to 1978 were given provisional marketing authorization until April 1990. At that time, manufacturers had to submit evidence of the safety and efficacy of the product according to the standards established by the Medicines Law of 1976.[4]

Commission E

In 1975, European Directive 75/319/EEC required member states to review the compliance of all medicinal products that were on the market at that time. The German Medicines Law of 1976 established a panel of experts to perform this review on herbal medicinal products.[5] The panel was called Commission E. It included physicians, pharmacists, nonmedical practitioners, pharmacologists, toxicologists, and pharmaceutical company representatives, all of whom were required to have training or clinical experience with herbal medicines. Similar to the American OTC review, Commission E reviewed active principles—rather than individual products—because of the huge number of products on the market and the enormity of the task.

Commission E was mandated to establish criteria for safety and efficacy, risk-benefit ratio of approval, and clear package labeling regarding possible risks. It based its evaluations primarily on information from the literature, experimental results, and the clinical experience of general practitioners. Data from clinical medical textbooks and evidence of traditional use were also considered. The Commission required all herbal medicinal products to be standardized using modern techniques.[6]

Commission E set pharmaceutical quality criteria for the active principles in over 300 medicinal plants. These plants comprised most of the ingredients found in industrially produced herbal medicinal products in Germany. The remaining products were reviewed one by one. In 1984, Commission E began publishing its findings as monographs in the *Federal Gazette (Bundesanzeiger)*. The next step was to review each "old" herbal medicinal product on the German market for compliance with the pharmaceutical quality criteria specified in the monographs.

Commission E monographs resulted in either a positive or negative risk-benefit assessment. Positive assessments granted marketing approval. These monographs detailed pharmacology, constituents, indications, side effects, contraindications, herb-drug interactions, dosages, mode of administration, duration of application, and activity in humans and animals. This information was distributed as package inserts with the herbal medicinal products. Negative assessment monographs stated the indication claimed by the manufacturer, the lack of supporting data, and the Commission's reasons for denying marketing approval.[7]

Commission E compiled its monographs between 1978 and 1994. It no longer has the authority to publish additional or updated monographs. However, the Commission E monographs are considered valid unless superseded by relevant new data, such as clinical trial results. The Commission now serves as an advisory board to the health authority. It is involved in the assessments of new and old herbal medicinal products.[8]

Old Products

The fifth amendment to the Medicines Law finalized the Commission E monographs (and the findings of all other commissions related to the drug review process). The fifth amendment permitted the ongoing sale of old products until December 31, 2004, if the reregistration application was withdrawn by December 31, 1995.[9] The sixth amendment to the Medicines Law extended the deadline to December 31, 1999. This provision was intended to help clear the backlog of old products. Manufacturers of these products bear the responsibility for them, and the documentation is not reviewed by the Federal Institute for Drugs and Medical Devices (BfArM, *Bundesinstitut für Arzneimittel und Medizinprodukte*). In 1994, this agency replaced the Federal Health Authority (BGA, *Bundesgesundheitsamt*). However, if a product is considered to endanger public health, it can be recalled.

In accordance with the fifth amendment to the Medicines Law,[10] the BfArM maintains a list of old products (marketed before 1978) for which proof of safety and efficacy is not required and for which particular traditional use claims are permitted. These products must reference a specific position on the list, have a claim for a mild indication (e.g., tonic), and be labeled "traditionally used." An expert commission determines which preparations and indications will be listed. It decides on the basis of documented evidence of the stated traditional use. Manufacturers choose whether to apply via this "traditional procedure." Many old herbal medicinal products lack scientific evidence of efficacy but can be approved through this alternative protocol. Unlike well-known new products, the manufacturer's evidence for quality is not reviewed. Also, the quality data need only comply with the earlier version of the Guidelines for Medicines Testing from December 14, 1989,[11] rather than the new version of May 5, 1995.[12]

New Products

All new medicinal products, including herbal medicinal products, are subject to the same requirements for proving quality, safety, and efficacy. There are two types of exceptions for medicinal products, which also apply to many herbal medicinal products: standardized marketing authorization and bibliographic evidence for well-known products.

Standardized Marketing Authorization

Under the Medicines Law, medicinal products that do not present a risk to the public's health may be exempted from premarket approval if they comply exactly with the standard marketing authorization monographs *(Standardzulassung)* published by the Ministry of Health. These monographs specify the quality, safety, and efficacy requirements, including analytical tests and text for labels and package inserts. Many such monographs have been published for herbal teas. Under this exemption, manufacturers are not required to submit any further documentation to the BfArM before marketing their products.

Bibliographic Proof for Well-Known Products

When a product is well known, as are many herbal medicines, the data on the quality of each product must still be submitted and approved. However, safety and efficacy can be proven with data from the literature ("bibliographic data").[13] Such data may be from pharmacology, toxicology, clinical, or observational studies, or from case reports and medical experience that have been scientifically evaluated and documented. Evidence for the safety and efficacy of herbal medicinal products is frequently drawn from Commission E monographs. If an early monograph is referenced, an updated literature review is also required.

Regardless of whether efficacy has been demonstrated with clinical studies, reference to an official monograph, or other data from the literature, only the specified indications are permissible as claims. For products marketed under a standardized marketing authorization, these indications may not be modified.

Many herbal medicinal products combine several botanical ingredients. Most of these products are well-known combinations of well-known ingredients and can be documented with data from the literature. However, if new ingredients are used or if a new combination of well-known ingredients is used, then a full application with complete data is required. For all combination products, each active ingredient must be shown to contribute to the overall product in compliance with the Medicines Law.[14] Additional guidance on combination products is provided in Assessment Criteria for Fixed Combinations, a working document by Commission E. It stipulates that each individual ingredient must contribute to the overall product's safety or efficacy by being efficacious, reducing side effects, or simplifying or improving the safety of the combination.

By 1998, Germany had authorized the sale of approximately 800 industrially produced finished herbal medicinal products. An additional 3,700 products were still undergoing review. This count does not include products that were exempted from premarket approval on the basis of compliance with standard marketing authorization monographs.

MANUFACTURING STANDARDS

Under the Medicines Law, the same manufacturing standards are applied to all medicinal products, including herbal medicinal products. Good manufacturing practices are spelled out in national legislation,[15] in accordance with European Directive 91/356/EEC. Inspections are carried out in Germany as well as in importing countries, such as China.

LABELING, ADVERTISING, DISTRIBUTION, AND RETAIL SALE

All medicinal products, including herbal medicinal products, are subject to the same labeling and advertising regulations.[16] New products must have package inserts. If there is no outer packaging, the label must include the information. Old products need to meet labeling requirements within one year of reregistration but most already comply.

Nonprescription drugs may be advertised to the general public in all media, with the exception of particular indications. Medical claims are not permitted for foods.[17] However, permitted health claims for foods include, for example, "helps maintain intestinal flora and supports resistance of the body" or "assists with control of cholesterol."[18] Misleading advertising, such as exaggerated claims[19] or presenting foods as medicines,[20] is prohibited.

In Germany, most herbal medicinal products are sold without a prescription and are covered by health insurance. Exclusions from coverage include particular indications, such as the common cold and laxatives, and certain substances, such as those that Commission E did not approve. Herbal medicinal products are sold in pharmacies. They may also be sold in a few other specific retail outlets, provided a qualified staff person is present during the sale. Those products that are not intended to treat illness, injury, aches, or pain may be sold outside pharmacies, including via mail order. Products approved under the traditional procedure may also be sold outside pharmacies.

Pharmacists may also sell herbal medicinal products that do not have marketing authorization if they meet one of the following conditions: (1) The product must be made for a particular person according to a prescription from a physician or practitioner *(Heilpraktiker)*. If the prescription is from a practitioner, the ingredients must be non-prescription substances.[21] (2) For products sold as prescription refills, batches of up to 100 packages per day may be prepared.[22]

POSTMARKET SAFETY AND SURVEILLANCE

The national surveillance system for medicinal products also monitors herbal medicinal products. Reports from consumers are accepted.

Several herbal medicinal products have been permanently withdrawn because of safety concerns. Others have been recalled then returned to the market after removing the harmful ingredients.

Chapter 5

France

LEGAL CLASSIFICATION

In France,[1] herbal products that are intended for medicinal use are regulated as drugs under the French Public Health Code.[2,3] This classification holds whether or not the active constituent is known. However, a single chemical compound that has been isolated from a plant is not classified as an herbal product.

Only pharmacists and qualified herbalists are permitted to sell herbal medicinal products.[4] The French Pharmacopoeia defines medicinal plants as those which have at least one part with medicinal properties.[5] Thus there is no legal classification for herbal medicinal products that lack prophylactic or therapeutic claims. However, in June 1979, new legislation authorized the retail sale of thirty-four herbals and seven herbal combinations.[6] Now these specific products may be sold as both drugs and beverages. Further legislation from September 1979 excludes widely used foods from use in pharmaceutical drugs.[7] With a few exceptions, selling herbal medicinal products that are mixed with pharmaceuticals, homeopathic ingredients, vitamins, or minerals is not permitted because separate approval is required for each category. There are a few exceptions that were already on the market before the legislation was enacted.

PROOF OF SAFETY AND EFFICACY

All medicinal products, including herbal medicinal products, require premarket approval[8] in line with government specifications.[9] The burden of proving the quality, safety, and efficacy of herbal medicinal products falls on the manufacturer. Medicinal products are defined by presentation (i.e., claims) and/or function.

Botanicals with traditional uses can be approved under an abridged procedure.[10] The French Medicines Agency *(Agence du Médicament)* maintains a "positive list" of approximately 200 herbal medicinal products that are recognized as having traditional uses for minor indications.[11] These botanicals were selected based on the pharmacological, toxicological, and/or clinical data in the literature, historical evidence of extensive traditional use, safety, a favorable risk-benefit ratio, chemical composition, and a well-established use for self-medication. General preparation protocols are given, and applicants must justify innovative preparations. A given herbal product can be marketed with a maximum of two indications. The indications are chosen from the positive list based on active constituents.

All botanicals that are not included on the positive list require a complete application. In all cases, chemical and pharmacological data are required. For some indications and herbal drugs (depending on the constituents), clinical data are also necessary. In general, bioavailability studies are not required. Requirements for toxicology data depend upon the preparation and constituents. Many herbal medicinal products require only an abbreviated set of toxicological data (Category 2) or none at all (Category 1). Others need to be tested as rigorously as any pharmaceutical drug. In principle, "bibliographic applications" based solely on data in the literature are accepted. However, to date, none of these applications has been approved.

For combination products that contain more than one botanical ingredient, only one set of data on the combination is required. Testing of the individual ingredients is not necessary. When justified, up to five ingredients from the positive list may be combined. For herbal teas, up to ten ingredients are allowed but only five may be considered the active constituents.

France has approved the sale of approximately 530 herbal medicinal products. Most have been authorized through the abridged protocol based on the positive list, rather than through a complete drug application. In recent years, there have been a handful of exceptions where full applications were needed, such as *Ginkgo biloba* (Tanakan), *Pygeum africanum* (Tadenan), and *Serenoa repens* (Permixon).

MANUFACTURING STANDARDS

The good manufacturing practices established by the European Union govern all drugs in France, including herbal medicinal products. When a "magisterial preparation" is prescribed by a physician to be prepared in the pharmacy, the pharmacist is responsible for ensuring the raw material used is pharmaceutical grade.

LABELING, ADVERTISING, DISTRIBUTION, AND RETAIL SALE

Since 1994, package inserts have been required for herbal medicinal products.[12] Other than laxatives, products that have been approved under an abridged procedure based on traditional uses are labeled "Traditionally used in . . ." (*"Traditionellement utilisé dans . . ."*)

With approval from the French Medicines Agency, medicines may be advertised to the general public in all types of media.[13] Medicines that are covered by insurance may not be advertised to the general public, but herbal medicinal products are generally not covered.

All medicinal products, including botanicals, are sold almost entirely in pharmacies.[14] Pharmacists are bound by a Code of Conduct that requires them to refrain from manufacturing, distributing, or selling any charlatan products.[15]

In principle, herbalists who hold a diploma are also permitted to sell botanicals, except products on the list of poisonous substances. Herbalists may sell combination products only if prepared after a consultation with a patient, except as authorized in legislation from 1943.[16] However, most botanicals are sold through pharmacies because the last diploma issued to an herbalist was in 1941 and few still practice.

POSTMARKET SAFETY AND SURVEILLANCE

National surveillance covers all approved medicinal products, including authorized botanicals. Monitoring relies on medical professionals voluntarily submitting adverse event reports. Package inserts instruct consumers to report adverse events to their physician or pharmacists. Except under extraordinary circumstances of severity or novelty, reports from consumers are not considered.

In 1992, herbal tea capsules that contained *Teucrium chamaedrys* (germandrée petit-chêne) were implicated in twenty-six reports of cytolitic hepatitis. Six herbal products were recalled as a result. They had been approved through an abridged procedure based on the positive list.

Herbal products are also sold in France illegally. For example, some products are bought through mail order or over the Internet. Monitoring of adverse events associated with these products is more problematic because consumers rarely tell their physicians about using an illegal product.

Chapter 6

United Kingdom

LEGAL CLASSIFICATION

In the United Kingdom,[1] herbal remedies that are industrially produced are regulated as drugs ("relevant medicinal products").[2] Herbal remedies were legally defined in 1968.[3] Some herbal remedies are exempt from premarket approval requirements. The classification "industrially produced" excludes botanicals that are manufactured or assembled in lockable premises (i.e., by a practitioner, who can be any person who gives advice on and makes herbal remedies, after a personal consultation) and then provided to a particular person in response to that person's request.[4] Plants that have been only dried, crushed, or comminuted and are labeled solely with the name of the plant are also excluded and may be sold through any retail outlet. If the writing on the label or package insert includes the name of the remedy or a recommended use, this exclusion does not apply.[5]

Certain products, such as peppermint and chamomile, are considered food unless a therapeutic claim is made on the label or package insert. In December 1995, the Medicines Control Agency (MCA) further clarified the distinction between herbal medicinal products, cosmetics, and foods.[6] Products containing mixtures of botanicals with vitamins and/or minerals are regulated as food supplements under food law. These products are not regulated as medicinal products as long as no therapeutic claims are made and MCA does not consider them to be medicinal based on function. If a botanical has a pharmacological effect at the recommended dose and has no use other than as a medicine, then MCA considers it to be medicinal based on function. MCA does not maintain a list of botanicals that are considered to be medicinal based on function, but examples include echinacea and St. John's wort.

PROOF OF SAFETY AND EFFICACY

All industrially produced medicinal products, including botanicals, require premarket approval through the same U.K. licensing system.[7] The burden of proving safety and efficacy falls on the manufacturer. Unlike in Germany and France, there is no abridged approval procedure in the United Kingdom. Either a botanical is completely exempt, or a full application is required. Exempt herbal remedies were discussed in the previous section. Other than these exceptions, new botanical products are held to the same standards of evidence and follow the same approval procedure as all other medicinal products. The requirements include complete clinical data.

Beginning in the 1970s, all medicinal products were granted a license of right which was subsequently reviewed to determine whether sufficient data had been provided. During this process, traditional use was considered for herbal medicines. Botanicals that were traditionally used and presented no safety concerns, were of satisfactory quality, and were indicated for minor self-limiting conditions were required to include the phrase "a traditional remedy for" in the labeling. This reference to traditional use continues to be required when these product licenses come up for renewal, but there are few such products still on the market.

Traditional use is not considered in new applications. However, new herbal medicines that are identical to products that have already been on the market for over ten years do not require proof of safety or efficacy. All other new botanical products need a complete application with clinical data. Proof of efficacy may be demonstrated with data from the literature on similar products ("bibliographic proof") if all requirements are met. The documents themselves (not just references) must be submitted, along with an English translation if needed, and an expert report. The challenge lies in determining what is a similar product.

By 1998, the United Kingdom had authorized the sale of 548 herbal medicine products. As of 1998, *Hypericum perforatum* L. (St. John's wort) and *Ginkgo biloba* L. had not been approved. (They require a full application. A depression claim for *Hypericum* would be a new clinical indication. *Ginkgo* would be considered a "new chemical entity.") In practice, several types of botanicals could be found on the market in the United Kingdom: (1) products exempt from pre-market approval because they are considered to be (a) foods, (b) food supplements that are nonmedicinal based on function and bear no therapeutic claim, (c) nonindustrially produced, (d) minimally processed and labeled only with the name of the plant; (2) grandfathered products identified on the label as "traditionally used for . . ."; (3) new products exempt from proving safety and efficacy because they are identical to old products; and (4) new products with full proof of safety and efficacy.

MANUFACTURING STANDARDS

Industrially produced herbal medicinal products are subject to the same good manufacturing practices (GMP) as all other medicinal products. Exempt herbal remedies are not covered by the GMP regulations.

LABELING, ADVERTISING, DISTRIBUTION, AND RETAIL SALE

Two amendments governing the labeling of packaging and package inserts were passed in 1992.[8,9] These U.K. statutes implemented the European Directive 92/27/EEC. The changes went into effect on January 1, 1994, for new products and at the time of license renewal for products already on the market. The main challenge in the implementation of the labeling regulations has been the ongoing inclusion of prohibited promotional information on labels. Exempt herbal remedies are not excluded from labeling regulations.

Advertising regulations for medicinal products also cover botanicals.[10,11,12] Medicinal products, including botanicals, may be sold to the public through pharmacies, other retail outlets, and mail order. General Sale List (GSL) medicines may be sold in manufacturers' sealed packaging from lockable premises—not necessarily a pharmacy. GSL medicines are generally sold in grocery stores, drugstores, and health food stores. Pharmacy medicine (P) and Prescription Only medicines (POM) may be sold only in a pharmacy.

In 1971, the Medicines Order granted some exemptions for botanicals from the usual licensing requirements applied to the sale, supply, and manufacture of medicinal products.[13] The exemptions were intended to permit herbalists to continue dispensing customized herbal medicines and to allow the retail sale of raw plant material. The exemptions from product authorization hold if the following conditions are met: no advertising is done; sale or supply is unsolicited; manufacture or assembly is under the supervision of staff qualified to ensure the product is of the character/specification required by the person; written records of the manufacture and sale are kept; a manufacturer's license is held.

In 1977, the Retail Sale or Supply of Herbal Remedies Order[14] further clarified retail sale and wholesale distribution. Botanicals listed in Part I of the Order can be sold only at a pharmacy. Herbal medicines listed in Parts II and III of the Order may be sold at a pharmacy or by practitioners to a particular person after a personal consultation. Only botanicals that have been dried, crushed, or comminuted may be sold without a sealed package from lockable premises—not necessarily a pharmacy.

POSTMARKET SAFETY AND SURVEILLANCE

Between 1992 and 1997, the Medical Toxicology Unit of Gruy's and St. Thomas's Hospital Trust conducted a study of adverse events associated with traditional remedies and dietary supplements. They concluded that most products do not endanger public safety. However, herbal products from China and India are a safety concern.

Since 1997, the surveillance system for adverse events (known as "adverse drug reactions" in the United Kingdom) has included herbal medicines. Package inserts instruct consumers to see their doctor or pharmacist if they experience ill effects. Official adverse event reports are accepted from physicians, dentists, coroners, and pharmacists, so that complaints can be verified and relevant medical histories reported. The Medicines Control Agency also requires manufacturers to report complaints that could be related to adverse events. Batches of herbal medicinal products have been recalled as a result of the monitoring system.

Chapter 7

Summary of International Regulatory Review

The regulation of botanicals has presented challenges for many countries. The regulatory systems in Canada, Germany, France, and the United Kingdom have been reviewed here because they are among the most refined and evolved. They serve to place the United States in the context of other industrialized nations that have grappled with the same issues and developed their own regulatory solutions. The principle features of the various systems are summarized in Table 7.1.

Each of these countries has made choices suited to its own culture, history, and needs. Although it would not be sensible for the United States to simply copy the system developed in another country, it is certainly possible that the United States could learn from the experience of other nations. Currently the United States is carving out a regulatory system that is unique in the world in its treatment of herbal medicinal products as dietary supplements that do not require premarket approval. Part IV of this book evaluates the limitations of this approach for protecting and promoting public health.

This brief international review of regulations would not be complete without mentioning the current harmonization efforts in Europe. Much work has been done but much also remains. In 1997, the European Commission and the European Agency for the Evaluation of Medicinal Products (EMEA) established the Ad Hoc Working Group on Herbal Medicinal Products to provide guidance on the harmonization process. This Working Group continues to play a key role. Each individual member state of the European Union has incorporated the relevant European Directives into their own national laws. The result has been disparate interpretations and implementations.

TABLE 7.1. Summary of Regulatory Situation for Botanicals in the United States, Canada, Germany, France, and United Kingdom

Country	Legal Classification	Burden of Proof	Premarket Approval Required	Simplified Approval for Traditional Use	Data from Scientific Literature Allowed	Number of Botanicals Approved
United States	dietary supplement	FDA	no	n/a	n/a	n/a
United States	OTC drug	manufacturer	yes	yes (in principle)	rule pending	fewer than 6
Canada (before)	food	manufacturer	no	n/a	n/a	n/a
Canada (before)	drug	manufacturer	yes[a]	yes	yes (in principle)	all but one are traditional
Canada (now)	natural health product	manufacturer	yes	yes	yes	—
Germany	medicinal product	manufacturer	yes[b]	yes	yes	800[c]
France	medicinal product	manufacturer	yes[d]	yes	yes (in principle)	530 (most are traditional)
United Kingdom	medicinal product	manufacturer	yes[e]	no	yes	548

Source: Adapted from Association of the European Self-Medication Industry (AESGP). 1998. Herbal medicinal products in the European Union. European Commission.
a Exempt if product is compounded or dispensed for a specific individual by a practitioner (including aboriginal healers). Exempt products may not contain restricted substances.
b Exempt if product is in compliance with official standard monographs.
c An additional 3,700 industrially produced herbal medicinal products were still undergoing review in Germany as of 1998. Also, this count does not include products that were exempted from premarket approval on the basis of compliance with official standard monographs.
d Exempt if product is one of thirty-four herbals and seven herbal combinations approved for sale as beverages.
e For exemptions, see Chapter 6.

98

In 1998, the European Commission selected the Association of the European Self-Medication Industry to conduct a review of the situation with herbal medicinal products in each of the fifteen member states. The resulting study is the most complete comparative review of European and North American regulations pertaining to herbal medicines. The report concluded that the most significant differences exist in the following areas: (1) classification of specific herbal products in various categories; (2) the option to acquire premarket approval on the basis of a full application, bibliographic application, or simplified proof of efficacy based on traditional use; and (3) retail distribution.[1] These disparities underscore the complexity of regulating herbal medicinal products. Although Europe is often held up as an example for the United States, it is important to remember that Europeans continue grappling with the issues raised by harmonization. Perhaps one of the key lessons the United States could learn from the European and Canadian experience is that they are making headway more quickly and efficiently because they treat herbal medicines as pharmacologically active substances. The result is a regulatory system for botanicals that is more effective at both protecting and promoting public health.

PART III:
ILLUSTRATIVE EXAMPLES

Chapter 8

Examples with Potential Public Health Benefits

ST. JOHN'S WORT AND MODERATE DEPRESSION

St. John's wort (*Hypericum perforatum* L.) was the first botanical selected by NIH to be the subject of a clinical trial. It is an example of an herbal medicine that could be an important treatment option for a highly prevalent disease. It also illustrates some of the research challenges presented by botanicals that are not encountered with pharmaceuticals. Most recently, it has begun to portend the risks of drug-herb interactions.

Depression afflicts over 17 million Americans annually and costs $44 billion in treatment, disability, and lost productivity (a cost similar to heart disease).[1,2] The number of pharmaceutical antidepressants available by prescription has grown rapidly over the past decade, however, "the problem of treating depression is far from solved despite the large number of drugs available."[3]

In Germany, products made from St. John's wort are commonly prescribed for the treatment of depression, and the cost is generally covered by health insurance. In contrast, in the United States, few physicians are even familiar with St. John's wort. Instead, consumer demand for St. John's wort has been driven more by word of mouth and the numerous articles that have appeared in the media, such as in *The New York Times*,[4,5] and in lay books.[6,7] In 1997, St. John's wort was the fifth most popular botanical on the U.S. market, capturing 6 percent of herbal supplement sales in all channels.[8] Growth in mass market sales was 20,000 percent.[9] Between 1995 and 1998, demand for the raw plant material of St. John's wort increased twelvefold from 500 tons per year to 6,000 tons per year, straining the available world supply of quality raw material.[10] Sales have since dropped off, falling 40 percent in 2001.[11] Judging from the media attention, sales figures, and lack of physician involvement, many Americans seem to be self-diagnosing and/or self-medicating their depression with St. John's wort products. If these products are not effective, the risk is that many of these cases of depression remain untreated. However, if St. John's wort is effective and safe (as it is understood to be in Germany), then it may offer a more cost-effective treatment with fewer side effects than pharmaceutical antidepressants.

In the case of antidepressants, producing fewer side effects is particularly important because patients who stop taking an antidepressant frequently do so because of the side effects they experience. In fact, the dropout rate is used in clinical studies as a measurement of side effects. In general, patients will stay on antidepressant medication longer if the side effects are less problematic. This means the benefits of the medicine are more likely to be seen and sustained over longer periods of time. Therefore, in addition to St. John's wort being an attractive treatment option at the individual level, there is an important and potentially very significant population-level advantage— that is, more patients staying on antidepressant treatment longer translates to greater improvement in the health status of the population as a whole.

The safety and efficacy of standardized extracts of St. John's wort have been widely studied in Germany.[12,13,14,15,16,17,18,19] Some studies have reported photosensitivity in animals after grazing on St. John's wort, but no published reports cite such phototoxicity in humans after oral administration of St. John's wort.[20] As of 1996, no reports of serious adverse consequences of any kind had been published in Germany.[21] However, since October 1999, several studies have suggested interactions between St. John's wort and certain prescription drugs. This concern has been particularly acute because of the high prevalence of St. John's wort use and because of the tendency of patients not to tell their physicians that they are taking it.

In October 1999, evidence of interactions between LI 160 (the St. John's wort product being tested by NIH) and digoxin were published.[22] On February 12, 2000, *The Lancet* published two letters on drug interactions with St. John's wort. The first reported on two patients who had rejected their heart transplants due to interactions between St. John's wort and cyclosporin.[23] The other was an NIH open label study of eight healthy volunteers taking indinavir (an anti-HIV protease inhibitor) and a St. John's wort product.[24] The investigators reported substantially decreased indinavir plasma concentrations, potentially due to induction of the cytochrome P450 metabolic pathway.

The FDA immediately issued an advisory notice regarding concurrent use of indinavir and other drugs with St. John's wort products.[25] They further advised that:

> St. John's wort may significantly decrease blood concentrations of all of the currently marketed HIV protease inhibitors (PIs) and possibly other drugs (to varying degrees) that are similarly metabolized, including the nonnucleoside reverse transcriptase inhibitors (NNRTIs). Consequently, concomitant use of St. John's wort with PIs or NNRTIs is not recommended because this may result in suboptimal antiretroviral drug concentrations, leading to loss of virologic response and development of resistance or class cross-resistance. . . . Based on this study and reports in the medical literature, St. John's wort appears to be an inducer of an important metabolic pathway, cytochrome P450. As many prescription drugs used to treat conditions such as heart disease, depression, seizures, certain cancers or to prevent conditions such as transplant rejection or pregnancy (oral contraceptives) are metabolized via this pathway, health care providers should alert patients about these potential drug interactions to prevent loss of therapeutic effect of any drug metabolized via the cytochrome P450 pathway.[26]

The active constituents and the mechanism of action of St. John's wort are not completely understood. Preliminary research indicated that an extract of St. John's wort inhibited the monoamine oxidase enzyme (MAO) in vitro.[27] However, subsequent studies showed that normal oral doses of St. John's wort were much too low to inhibit MAO in vivo.[28] In practice, MAO-inhibitor type side effects have never been observed with St. John's wort.[29] More recently, research on the mechanism of action of St. John's wort has focused on serotonin.[30,31,32] Until recently the polycyclic phenols hypericin and pseudohypericin were thought to be the major active constituents.

However, recent data suggest that hyperforin is the key constituent involved in reuptake.[33,34,35,36,37,38,39] This is a typical profile for an herbal medicine, where multiple compounds in the mixture contribute to the efficacy and it is not possible to attribute the biological activity to a single compound. The importance of human data becomes especially relevant because of this chemical complexity.

When NIH was evaluating the proposal for a U.S. clinical trial on St. John's wort and depression it was particularly compelled by one meta-analysis.[40] In this 1996 study, twenty-three randomized clinical trials (most conducted in Germany) were selected from the literature and evaluated for methodological quality. The trials included a total of 1,757 outpatients diagnosed with mild or moderate depression and treated with one of several formulations of St. John's wort for four to eight weeks. Fifteen of the studies compared the efficacy of the St. John's wort formulation to placebo and eight trials compared it to an antidepressive drug therapy. In the meta-analysis, efficacy results were pooled to estimate the responder rate ratio, which is responder rate in treatment group divided by responder rate in the control group. To evaluate side effects, dropouts were tabulated. The researchers concluded that St. John's wort may be useful for the treatment of mild to moderate depression, is superior to placebo, and has fewer side effects than standard antidepressants. However, the conclusions of the meta-analysis were limited by the heterogeneity among studies in diagnoses, doses, formulations, and blinding, and the short duration of all twenty-three clinical trials.

In October 1997, NIH began funding a $4.3 million, thirteen-center clinical trial on a German St. John's wort product (LI 160) for moderately severe depression—not mild to moderate depression as suggested by the British meta-analysis just described. The NIH study included 340 patients in three treatment groups, each of whom received one of the following: (1) a standardized 900 mg to 1,500 mg dose of LI 160; (2) a 50 mg to 100 mg dose of sertraline (Zoloft), which is a selective serotonin reuptake inhibitor (SSRI) and a leading pharmaceutical antidepressant; or (3) placebo. The treatment period was longer than in previous studies. It included an eight-week controlled period and eighteen weeks of follow-up.

The results of this major study were published in the *Journal of the American Medical Association* (*JAMA*) in April 2002 and showed both St. John's wort and Zoloft to be ineffective as compared to placebo for moderately severe depression in this trial. A full response to treatment was seen in 31.9 percent of patients who received the placebo, 24.8 percent of patients who took Zoloft, and 23.9 percent of those treated with St. John's wort. On a secondary measure, Zoloft scored better than the placebo.[41]

The lack of efficacy seen in Zoloft, which is a widely used FDA-approved pharmaceutical antidepressant, underscores the challenges of this type of research. Even a gold standard randomized, double-blind, controlled clinical intervention trial can yield perplexing results. Zoloft was included in the study design not for comparison with St. John's wort but rather as a positive control to aid the interpretation of just this kind of result. In their *JAMA* report, the researchers point out that without a placebo treatment group in this study, the results would have suggested that St. John's wort and Zoloft were equally effective. If there had been no Zoloft treatment group, then the outcome would have implied St. John's wort was ineffective. However, because Zoloft was also ineffective in this study, the researchers note that the possibility must be considered that the assay was not sufficiently sensitive to detect the effects of either treatment. It is also critical to underscore that St. John's wort is generally considered to be a treatment for mild to moderate depression, and not for moderately severe depression. This would be another reasonable explanation for the inefficacy seen in St. John's wort in this trial. As the researchers state in their *JAMA* report "Hypericum may be most effective in less severe major depression . . . but further study of this possibility needs to be conducted. . . ." [42]

Until such an investigation is conducted, the question of efficacy will remain open. In the absence of such evidence, medical professionals are unlikely to familiarize themselves with LI 160 as a treatment option or advise their patients on the use of LI 160 as an alternative. Meanwhile, many consumers are probably going to continue to self-medicate with St. John's wort products, often without telling their physicians, and the risks associated with this approach will persist.

Ideally, a future study would include a cost-effectiveness component. If, for example, St. John's wort turns out to be somewhat less effective than sertraline, a cost-effectiveness analysis would be warranted. Such an evaluation would weigh the cost of treatment against the improvement in quality of life. It might consider factors such as the considerably lower cost of St. John's wort, the lesser side effects, and the concomitant willingness for patients to remain on the medication for longer periods of time. It is certainly still plausible that St. John's wort, when taken as a monotherapy, could turn out to be a more cost-effective treatment option than pharmaceuticals in some cases of mild to moderate depression.

GINKGO AND ALZHEIMER'S DISEASE

Ginkgo biloba L. is the second herbal medicine the NIH has chosen to be the subject of a clinical trial. Alzheimer's disease is a growing public health concern because the population in the age groups at risk is increasing. Approximately 1.5 million people now have severe Alzheimer's disease and 7.5 million are projected to have it by 2040. The use of pharmaceutical treatments for Alzheimer's disease is limited because of their severe side effects. Extracts of *Ginkgo biloba* L. standardized at 24 percent ginkgo flavoneglycosides are rapidly becoming an attractive treatment option in the United States. When taken during the early stages of the disease, these extracts appear to reverse or slow the progression of the disease.[43,44,45,46]

Ginkgo has been widely used in Europe and in the Far East for many years. There are over 400 articles in the medical literature on *Ginkgo biloba* L. A 1992 Dutch review of forty human studies of ginkgo concluded that ginkgo causes no serious side effects.[47] The absence of side effects is particularly important for ginkgo because it means the treatment can be continued uninterrupted for the rest of a patient's life. As with St. John's wort, the absence of side effects also means people are more likely to actually take the medicine over a long period of time. If high quality ginkgo products were widely available in the United States and medical professionals and the elderly were informed about it, improvements in the prevalence of Alzheimer's might be possible.

In the same Dutch study just cited, ginkgo was also found to be as effective as codergocrine, a widely prescribed pharmaceutical at that time. The effectiveness of ginkgo versus placebo in the early stages of Alzheimer's disease was further demonstrated in two clinical trials published in 1997.[48] The second study[49] was published in the *Journal of the American Medical Association*'s (*JAMA*'s) special issue on aging. It was the first U.S. placebo-controlled, double-blind, randomized clinical trial on an extract of *Ginkgo biloba* L. for dementia. In that trial, no major side effects were reported. The disease was stabilized and in 64 percent of the patients mental function improved.

Dr. Turan Itil is a neuropsychiatrist and a co-author of the *JAMA* article. He is a world authority on the pharmacology of the brain, a leader in the development of pharmaceutical treatments for brain diseases, and chairman of the World Health Organization's International Advisory Committee on the Diagnosis, Prevention, and Treatment of Alzheimer's Disease. Dr. Itil takes ginkgo to protect his memory; so do his wife and "most of my friends over age sixty-five,"[50] he says. He is also recommending worldwide clinical trials on *Ginkgo biloba* L. because the evidence is so compelling and the need is so great.[51]

In September 1999, NIH granted funding for a six-year, $15 million multicenter trial on *Ginkgo biloba* L. for Alzheimer's disease. The study will include 2,000 patients in two treatment groups: (1) 240 mg of standardized ginkgo extract; and (2) placebo. Patients will be closely monitored for side effects. There are concerns about possible bleeding when ginkgo is taken concurrently with aspirin; interactions with drugs are always a concern with botanicals. With ginkgo it is particularly important that research addresses possible drug-botanical interactions because ginkgo is taken by elderly people. This population typically uses multiple pharmaceuticals concurrently.

ECHINACEA AND THE COMMON COLD

One of the ironies of allopathic medicine is that despite its heroic accomplishments it has little to offer for the treatment of the common cold. If cold symptoms are due to a bacterial infection, antibiotics may help. However, if the infectious agent is viral, there is no pharmaceutical treatment (other than for alleviation of the symptoms). In this example, an herbal medicine for the common cold is presented as a third botanical with potential benefit for public health. The NIH, so far, has not funded a clinical trial on this plant, but the Center for Dietary Supplements Research at the University of California in Los

Angeles has received NIH support to conduct pilot research on the specific immune enhancing actions of echinacea.

The genus *Echinacea* is native to the American plains. Several species are used medicinally: *E. purpurea* (L.) Moench., *Echinacea angustifolia* D.C. var. angustifolia, and *E. pallida* (Nutt.) Nutt. There are numerous common names; the one that is used most often is purple coneflower. Echinacea was taken as a medicine by Native Americans. It was introduced into U.S. allopathic medicine in 1887 and was widely taken to treat cold and flu for about four decades.[52] In Germany, echinacea has been used for decades and is approved as an over-the-counter drug for boosting the immune system and fighting respiratory and urinary tract infections. In 1994, Germans received over 2.5 million prescriptions for echinacea to treat the common cold.[53] Echinacea has been the most popular botanical sold in the United States since 1995.[54]

The activity of echinacea is primarily on the nonspecific cellular immune system.[55] Two studies in particular have supported the use of *Echinacea purpurea* (L.) Moench. for treating colds.[56,57] One more recent trial on *E. angustifolia* and *E. purpurea* did not observe a prophylactic effect against upper respiratory tract infection.[58] A 1994 review of echinacea evaluated twenty-six clinical trials.[59] The researchers concluded that several studies clearly demonstrated that echinacea has immune-stimulating and infection-fighting properties, especially against upper respiratory tract infections. However, the review was inconclusive on the optimum echinacea preparation and dose. A 1996 review article on echinacea pointed out that results vary depending on the species, part of the plant, and preparation used.[60] This principle is generally true for herbal medicines.

The taxonomic history of echinacea illustrates another type of complexity involved in herbal medicine research that does not come up with pharmaceuticals. Prior to 1968, the two species that are now called *Echinacea angustifolia* and *Echinacea pallida* were considered to be one and the same species. The genus *Echinacea* was revised in 1968,[61] but these types of taxonomic changes take time to become widely used. As a result, it is now suspected that prior to 1987 a substantial amount of commercial *"Echinacea angustifolia"* was actually *Echinacea pallida*. This introduces ambiguity into the interpretation of the scientific literature on echinacea from that period. It also underscores the importance of tight botanical quality control and the importance of archiving botanical specimens from each production lot for identification purposes. The consequences of poor botanical quality control come up again in the adulteration example presented in Chapter 9.

Chapter 9

Examples That Present Public Health Risks

EPHEDRA

Ephedra is a prominent example of the FDA attempting to take regulatory action in response to adverse event reports. It illustrates a situation in which the FDA's efforts at enforcement have been ineffective. *Ephedra* refers to a variety of herbal products that contain ephedrine alkaloids. The ingredients in these products are commonly known as ma huang, ephedra, Chinese ephedra, and epitonin, and primarily include the species *Ephedra sinica* Stapf, *E. equistestina* Bunge, *E. intermedia* var. *tibetica* Stapf, and *E. distachya* L. Two billion doses of botanical ephedrine alkaloids are consumed in the United States annually. The FDA has received more adverse event reports on ephedra than on any other botanical. There are currently over 1,000 adverse event reports listed on the FDA Web site that contain the words *ephedra, ephedrine,* or *ma huang.* The FDA's disclaimer on these reports notes, among other points, that: (1) these descriptions are presented exactly as they were submitted (except where summaries of overly technical language were needed); and (2) there is no way to ascertain from these reports whether the implicated agent actually caused the adverse event.

In the *Federal Register* dated June 4, 1997, after weighing its regulatory options and the limitations of the available data, the FDA concluded that without premarket review authority they could not ban ephedra products from the market. However, the FDA did issue a proposed rule to limit the allowable dose of ephedrine alkaloids in botanical products to 8 mg per serving.[1] These restrictions were based on the FDA's authority under DSHEA. Under that provision, the FDA is permitted to take enforcement action when it can prove that a product may present a significant or unreasonable risk of illness or injury when it is used as directed on the label or, in the absence of labeling, under conditions of ordinary use. The comment period for this proposed rule closed on December 2, 1997.

In July 1999, the U.S. General Accounting Office (GAO) issued its response to the FDA's proposed rule.[2] It questioned the basis for the FDA's conclusions about causation and the proposed dose. The GAO pointed out that even by the FDA's own account, the passive adverse event reports that the FDA had cited often lacked information on the product identification, doses ingested, duration of use, and medical diagnoses. The scientific data on dosage of ephedrine alkaloids are also incomplete. The FDA's final rule on ephedra is pending.

Meanwhile, the Federal Trade Commission has taken regulatory action on alleged misrepresentations in the advertising of the herbal product called "Herbal Ecstasy," which contains ephedrine alkaloids. Also, legislation on ephedra has been proposed independently in several states (Texas, California, Indiana, Virginia, Vermont, Illinois, Hawaii, Iowa, New York, New Hampshire, Montana, Pennsylvania, and Massachusetts). Proposals have ranged from a complete ban on ephedra (in Texas, rejected) to exempting dietary supplements from the law that restricts over-the-counter sale of ephedrine products (in Montana).[3] In May 1998, the Texas Department of Health indicated that since 1993 they had received 1,200 reports of adverse effects associated with ephedra. On May 15, 1998, the Texas Board of Health approved rules to classify ephedrine as a dangerous drug and to require prescriptions for dietary supplements containing ephedrine.[4]

In 1998, the first lawsuit over ephedra went to trial when a woman sued the manufacturer of a weight loss dietary supplement called AMP II, which contains ephedrine and caffeine.[5] The plaintiff claimed that the stroke she had suffered three years earlier at the age of thirty-four had been caused by AMP II. She had been taking drops of AMP II in her coffee three times a day for nearly two years when the stroke occurred. According to testimony in the trial, the manufacturer's revenue on AMP II had peaked at $50 million a year, and the company founder had earned up to $10 million annually. The jury ruled ten to two in favor of the manufacturer.

In December 2000, *The New England Journal of Medicine* (*NEJM*) published an FDA-commissioned study of adverse event reports on ephedra.[6] Of 140 reports evaluated, 31 percent were found to be definitely or probably associated with the use of ephedra and another 31 percent were considered to be possibly linked to ephedra. Among the reports that were definitely, probably, or possibly related to ephedra, there were ten deaths and thirteen permanent disabilities. The adverse events reported included hypertension, palpitations, tachycardia, stroke, and seizures.

In 2001, the judged ordered a retrial of the AMP II case, based on new evidence that had been released by the FDA under the Freedom of Information Act.[7] The *NEJM* study described previously was also submitted as evidence. This time, the jury voted eleven to one in favor of the plaintiff and awarded her $13.3 million—$1.3 million for medical bills and $12 million in punitive damages. The judge later reduced the total to $13.1 million. The manufacturer has since appealed. Meanwhile, the FDA seized the company's inventory of AMP II, and the firm has ceased selling AMP II. However, it has continued to market other products that contain ephedrine and caffeine and maintains that its products are safe.

In November 1997, the President's Commission on Dietary Supplement Labels had urged the FDA to take action on ephedra. By September 2001, the National Football League, the National Collegiate Athletic Association, and the International Olympic Committee had all banned the use of ephedrine.[8] The scientific and regulatory debate over ephedra continue.

ADULTERATION CASE REPORT

In contrast to the ephedra situation, in the following example, the FDA was able to respond effectively to an adverse event report. In May 1997, the FDA received a report of a twenty-three-year-old woman who had been admitted to the hospital after ingesting an herbal "cleansing" program comprised of five dietary supplement products. She presented with nausea, vomiting, dizziness, irregular heart rate with heart block, and toxic levels of digoxin. One month later, the FDA received a second adverse event report very similar to the first. The implicated product contained fourteen botanicals. The FDA applied sophisticated chemical analyses and conducted challenging taxonomic identifications from pulverized plant material.

After a thorough investigation, they found *Plantago lanceolata* L. (plantain) was the ingredient adulterated with *Digitalis lanata* Ehrh.

On June 12, 1997, the FDA issued a statement warning that some dietary supplement products labeled as containing "plantain" might be contaminated with *Digitalis lanata* Ehrh. At the time the contamination was confirmed, 7 million tablets had been ready to ship and were recalled. The FDA's trace to suppliers involved approximately 6,000 pounds of adulterated plantain that had been distributed over a period of two and a half years. Fifteen companies, including several hundred establishments and individuals, received recall actions. No known deaths resulted from this incident. This example demonstrates the gaps in quality control of botanicals and the severity of the associated public health risks. A letter in *The New England Journal of Medicine* further pointed out that "the unavailability of assays for laboratory analysis compounds the problem of the dearth of pre- and post-marketing data on toxicity."[9]

COMFREY

Comfrey (*Symphytum officinale* L.) is an example of an herbal product that has been restricted in Germany and Canada but remains on the market in the United States. Comfrey contains pyrrolizidine alkaloids that have been linked to veno-occlusive disease and liver tumors in humans.[10] In Germany, the use of comfrey has been restricted to the external use of the root with a limit on the pyrrolizidine alkaloid content. In the United States, comfrey remains available in some health food stores and via mail order and the Internet, although it is sold less widely than in previous years. In July 1996, the American Herbal Products Association, a trade organization representing the dietary supplement industry, began recommending that manufacturers include the following warning on products containing comfrey: "For external use only. Do not apply to broken or abraded skin. Do not take while nursing." Many manufacturers voluntarily include such warnings or have removed comfrey from their products. However, this warning is not required to be on the label and in the United States it is still quite possible for a consumer to obtain comfrey without being aware of the serious risks associated with it.

On July 6, 2001, the FDA sent a letter to eight trade associations representing the botanical dietary supplement industry advising manufacturers to remove comfrey products from the market. It stated that the scientific evidence was sufficient for the FDA to consider products that contain comfrey or other sources of pyrrolizidine alkaloids to be adulterated under the Federal Food, Drug, and Cosmetic Act and that the FDA was prepared to use its authority and resources to remove these products from the market. In tandem, the Federal Trade Commission (FTC) took action against two companies that were marketing comfrey-containing products. Both firms agreed to injunctions prohibiting them from marketing these products for internal use or for use on open wounds, and requiring the following warning on the label of products sold for external use:

> WARNING: External Use Only. Consuming this product can cause serious liver damage. This product contains comfrey. Comfrey contains pyrrolizidine alkaloids, which may cause serious illness or death. This product should not be taken orally, used as a suppository, or applied to broken skin. For further information contact the Food and Drug Administration: http//vm.cfsan.fda.gov

Perhaps these actions will deter others from selling comfrey-containing products intended for ingestion. If not, the FDA and/or the FTC will have the costly task of identifying these products and taking action on a case-by-case basis.

PART IV:
ANALYSIS OF CURRENT
AND POTENTIAL IMPACT
ON PUBLIC HEALTH

Chapter 10

Safety

Chapters 10 through 14 argue that the current regulatory and business environments constrain the potential benefits of botanicals as well as the protection from risk. In 1997, 12.1 percent of American adults had used at least one herbal medicine in the previous twelve months.[1] Sales continued to rise in 1998,[2] began to plateau in 1999, and remained flat in 2000.[3] The increase in use and in available products places the American population at greater risk. Meanwhile, the benefits Americans receive from herbal medicines are attenuated by many factors. Part IV discusses these issues.

Safety was a frequent topic during the congressional debates that led up to the Dietary Supplement Health and Education Act of 1994 (DSHEA). In general, consumers tend to believe herbs are safe because these products are natural and are sold over the counter without a prescription. The President's Commission on Dietary Supplement Labels indicated that although many herbs are quite safe under normal use, there are some (e.g., ephedra) which raise concerns about safety. As the examples described in the previous section illustrate, the risks in some cases can be life threatening. One of the most egregious shortcomings of the current situation with botanicals in the United States is the extreme difficulty in distinguishing the numerous safe herbal products from the few that are unsafe. This section analyzes the situation in two parts: (1) safety issues related to the absence of premarket approval; (2) the limitations of current postmarket surveillance.

ABSENCE OF PREMARKET APPROVAL

The United States is unique among industrialized nations in not requiring premarket approval of herbal medicines. However, the Dietary Supplement Health and Education Act of 1994 (DSHEA) does have some premarket provisions in the form of notification letters, good manufacturing practices, new dietary ingredients, and labeling.

Notification Letters

DSHEA requires that a manufacturer notify the FDA about a structure/function label claim within the first thirty days after a product launch. The President's Commission suggested that the documentation substantiating the claim also include evidence of safety. However, there are several major limitations to the effectiveness of this procedure in protecting public safety. First, the contents of the manufacturer's substantiation file—including evidence of safety—are not specified by DSHEA. The President's Commission provided suggestions for substantiation files but rule making was not revisited to officially incorporate these suggestions as requirements. Evidence of safety is therefore prudent for a manufacturer to have—but not required.

Second, the product may be marketed with or without the concurrence of the FDA. The burden of proving the existence of a risk falls on the FDA. Under DSHEA, the FDA is not obliged to prove that harm has actually occurred, only that a "significant or unreasonable risk of illness or injury" exists.[4] Supplement proponents claim that this language represents a tougher standard than the one for food (where the FDA must show that an injury has actually occurred). However, in practice little research is done on botanicals, so data are scarce, and the basis for establishing a "significant or unreasonable risk of illness or injury"[5] is limited. Again, the case of ephedra illustrates this point well. The FDA is apparently not equipped with the resources or the infrastructure to thoroughly evaluate every letter of notification.

Good Manufacturing Practices

In 1994, Section 9 of DSHEA extended the application of existing good manufacturing practices (GMPs) to include dietary supplements. DSHEA also allows for the development of additional GMP regulations specifically for dietary supplements. So far, during the subsequent five years, industry submitted draft GMP regulations; the FDA reviewed the draft, issued a proposed rule, formed a Working

Group of the Food Advisory Committee, and in July 1999 began a series of public meetings on this topic. Setting standards for an industry with such a diverse array of products is clearly an enormous undertaking. The FDA has indicated it will issue a proposed rule on dietary supplement GMPs in FY2002, accept comments, and issue its final rule in FY2003. In the meantime, botanical product quality control standards vary widely. Chemical composition varies among products from the same species and among bottles of the same product from the same manufacturer. Even the best informed consumers and professionals struggle to distinguish among quality, mediocre, and dangerous products and/or doses.

New Dietary Ingredients

Section 8 of DSHEA provides specific requirements for premarket FDA notification of "new dietary ingredients." These are defined as ingredients that were first sold on the U.S. market after October 15, 1994. DSHEA requires the manufacturer to demonstrate that the new dietary ingredient can "reasonably be expected to be safe." The manufacturer must submit all evidence at least seventy-five days before the product enters interstate commerce. The FDA may prohibit marketing if they are not satisfied with the evidence, but premarket authorization is not required. Ninety days after receipt, the FDA must place the nonproprietary information provided by the manufacturer on public display.

The procedure for new dietary ingredients is the most thorough one mandated by DSHEA. In principle it would allow the FDA to prevent hazardous new ingredients from entering the U.S. market. However, in practice, it does little to protect public safety for several reasons. First, relatively few herbal medicines on the U.S. market are new. As shown in Chapter 14, the top twenty botanicals comprise 62 percent of sales. Second, the FDA estimates that a manufacturer will spend only twenty hours extracting and summarizing the necessary data from its files. Industry did not dispute this estimate. Such a brief report will probably not contain very substantial data. Furthermore, it is likely the data will be derived from public sources rather than from original research conducted by the manufacturer (for reasons discussed in the next chapter). As such, the data may or may not be truly relevant to the product in question. Third, the acceptable safety standards for a new dietary ingredient are ambiguous. It is unclear whether a history of use in other countries will constitute valid evidence of safety. The precise nature of the evidence that is required is also vague. Overall, although DSHEA's provisions for new dietary ingredients would, in principle, contribute to the protection of public health, in practice they have minimal impact.

Labeling

Other than structure/function claims (discussed in Chapter 13), U.S. botanical labeling discussions have focused on complete and accurate disclosure of ingredients and nutrient content. The result has been changes in labeling requirements that have cost manufacturers enormous sums to implement. In the end, no one benefited from these changes and they had little or no impact on the safety of herbal medicine products. Consumers are not taking botanicals for their nutrient content. They are generally seeking a pharmacological effect, however subtle. The time, effort, and resources spent on nutrient labeling could have been far better invested. For example, labels should bear warnings about known drug-botanical interactions.

POSTMARKET SURVEILLANCE

In the absence of premarket approval, the importance of postmarket surveillance is amplified. The adulteration example in Chapter 9 showed that there are numerous points in the supply chain where contamination may occur. These loopholes also make postmarket monitoring critical. However, in the United States, postmarket surveillance of adverse events is done only passively. As illustrated in the ephedra example in Chapter 9 and substantiated by the inspector general's study[6] described in Chapter 2, adverse event reports are frequently incomplete, making causality extremely difficult to investigate. The findings reported by the inspector general indicate that a cooperative surveillance system for botanicals is far from being realized: the FDA is not properly disclosing adverse event reports and manufacturers are submitting very few adverse event reports to the FDA (fewer than ten between 1994 and 1999), product samples are often not provided when requested, and even the city and state of the manufacturer in many cases cannot be found. Further, since there is no legal requirement to submit adverse event reports, it is quite possible that many events are never reported to the surveillance databases.

The ephedra example also demonstrates that the FDA does not have the resources to conduct the necessary research on even the most problematic botanicals. Under these circumstances, it is highly improbable that chronic toxicity, such as liver toxicity, would be identified. Also, with inadequate data, enforcement is problematic. The President's Commission pointed out that "The apparent safety of the majority of products now marketed as dietary supplements actually increases the importance of having adequate enforcement mechanisms, because consumers may then assume that a wide margin of safety automatically applies to any product classified as a dietary supplement."[7]

All these considerations underscore the need for a postmarket surveillance system that can quickly identify high-risk botanicals and effectively take action to protect consumer health. Acknowledging the high-risk profile of particular products need not cast doubt or suspicion on botanicals in general.

Chapter 11

Research

Although millions of Americans are consuming herbal medicines, very few of these products have undergone rigorous preclinical or clinical trials to optimize product standardization, dosage, formulation, and treatment regimens, nor have they been the subject of epidemiological study. Many of the public health issues with botanicals in the United States relate to the paucity of research. This section explores the constraints on research.

PATENT PROTECTION

Botanicals tend to be natural or generic products without substantial human innovation involved, which makes patenting difficult.[1] Also, U.S. patent law for pharmaceuticals is based almost exclusively on pure molecular entities. The fact that botanicals often contain complex mixtures of compounds and multiple active constituents further complicates patenting. The lack of patent protection for herbal medicine products is a major barrier to the funding of U.S. research by manufacturers. In turn, the constraints on research limit the available data.

It is a useful thought experiment to consider what the consequences might be if a U.S. manufacturer were able to patent its product. For example, the patent might be based on a unique manufacturing process. Protected by a patent, the manufacturer could then justify a substantial investment in preclinical and clinical studies. After generating sufficient data from these studies, and perhaps identifying the active constituent(s), it might then be possible to attain over-the-counter drug status for the product. As an OTC drug, medical professionals might be more comfortable recommending its use for a specified indication. More patients would learn about the availability of the product and more would be inclined to try an herbal medicine if recommended by their physician. The botanical would thus become more widely available to those in need. If the herbal medicine cost less than its pharmaceutical counterpart, the individual would save money. If the botanical had fewer side effects, then the patient might be more inclined to continue using it. This would be particularly true if the product treated a chronic condition. With this new market opportunity, the manufacturer might be well rewarded for investing in research. Overall, the result might be an additional treatment option at a lower cost with fewer side effects. Although this scenario may seem to be conjecture in the United States, it is commonplace in other industrialized countries.

PRODUCT-SPECIFIC RESEARCH
BY MANUFACTURERS

Without patent protection, U.S. manufacturers are not inclined to conduct research on the safety and efficacy of their products because it would not be profitable. As is evident in the pharmaceutical industry, such research is extremely expensive. If a U.S. manufacturer of herbal medicines were to fund research on its products, there would be little to prevent its competitors from using the resulting data for their own purposes. Under these circumstances, manufacturers actually have a disincentive to conduct or fund research. This situation is unfortunate because research is badly needed on herbal medicines, and these for-profit producers of botanicals are capable of bearing most of the cost of research, as the pharmaceutical industry does. Botanical manufacturers are reaping profits without funding research and the public may be paying the price.

One possible solution to this fundamental problem would be to require product-specific data. Then patenting would become less relevant and manufacturers would have an incentive to conduct research on their products. The Nutraceuticals Research and Education Act drew on this concept. (NREA is discussed at the end of Chapter 2.) The FDA's proposed rule on OTC botanicals addresses this problem by providing a three-year period of exclusivity for unpatented products. However, it is unclear whether an exclusivity period of three years will be a sufficient incentive for manufacturers to invest in research.

Premarketing letters of notification do not require FDA approval, nor do they stipulate that there must be data in the manufacturer's substantiation file on its specific product. Consequently manufacturers have little reason to conduct their own research and a large incentive to "borrow science" from the literature and other products for their own substantiation files. Data from these public sources may or may not be relevant to their own products. Furthermore, much of the available data comes from studies in Europe, where patenting is more common. At least one European manufacturer has issued a warning in the United States about borrowing their science. Willmar Schwabe indicated that it will be enforcing its U.S. patent rights over its formulation of *Ginkgo biloba* L.[2] (Schwabe's product was used in the study published in the *Journal of the American Medical Association* on dementia.)[3]

GOVERNMENT RESEARCH FUNDING

For the reasons just discussed, research funding for herbal medicine is very limited in the United States. As a result, much of the publicly available data come from other countries and are not currently applicable under U.S. law. In addition, most American physicians do not read foreign medical journals, particularly if they are not written in English. American physicians also have a tendency to consider foreign medical journals and research to be of inferior scientific quality, whether or not this is objectively the case. For these reasons, most American physicians are not aware of the body of research conducted on herbal medicines in other countries.

Recently, U.S. government research funding has begun to increase. In October 1997, the National Institutes of Health (NIH) funded a three-year, $4.3 million, multicenter clinical trial on St. John's wort for moderate depression. In September 1999, NIH sponsored a six-year, $15 million trial on *Ginkgo biloba* L. for dementia. In October 1999, NIH established two Dietary Supplement Research Centers to investigate the biological effects of botanicals. The University of Illinois in Chicago and the University of California in Los Angeles each received a grant of $1.5 million annually for five years.

According to NIH, its reasons for these initiatives were: (1) botanicals are widely used for primary health care in developing countries; (2) botanicals are regulated and prescribed as drugs in Germany; and (3) millions of Americans are using botanicals.

Congress appropriated year 2000 and 2001 funds for additional Dietary Supplement Research Centers and the NIH Office of Dietary Supplements (ODS) has continued to award grants. The corresponding press release stated "The creation of such Centers is needed to advance the quality and quantity of scientific information on botanicals and to promote further research in this area."[4] The creation of the National Center for Complementary and Alternative Medicine (NCCAM) and the White House Commission on Complementary and Alternative Medicine Policy bode well for ongoing research funding that may sometimes include botanicals. For example, in 2001, NCCAM committed approximately $4.3 million for fifteen grants to support studies on drug-botanical interactions.

EPIDEMIOLOGICAL RESEARCH

The U.S. situation with botanicals is ideally suited for observational studies. Millions of people are already consuming these products, so there are enormous opportunities for gathering observational human data. Concurrently, millions of others are choosing not to take botanicals who could be included in comparison groups.

As pointed out by the President's Commission, the vast majority of botanicals are safe. For those products that are considered safe, it is not necessary to go back to preclinical in vitro and in vivo studies. Because herbal medicines tend to be complex chemically and mechanisms of action often involve multiple compounds, the best way to understand their effect on humans is often through human studies. Although intervention trials are the gold standard ideal, they are also very expensive and therefore not feasible for all products. Well-designed observational studies would be the next best option and perhaps more powerful than low-budget clinical studies with small sample sizes. Opportunities to gather large epidemiological human data sets on herbal medicines abound because these products are widely used. Sound epidemiological data would contribute greatly to a better understanding of the public health impact of the current regulatory situation with botanicals in the United States and would powerfully enhance the current passive surveillance system.

Study designs should allow detection of both acute and chronic toxicity, as well as therapeutic benefits. There is a notable absence of a coordinated effort to gather high-quality observational data to monitor and systematically evaluate the *beneficial* effects of botanicals. The potential power of such a data set would be particularly significant for some of the most commonly used botanicals consumed by millions of Americans. Herbal medicines taken to treat chronic diseases would also be high priorities for epidemiological studies because of the importance of understanding their effects over a long period of time. Primarily manufacturers should fund these studies, but there are many possibilities for collaboration.

As formularies* begin to include herbal medicine products, a new opportunity for data collection may emerge. In order for a product to be included in a formulary, manufacturers could be required to conduct clinical trials, systematically gather epidemiological data on safety and efficacy, and submit complete adverse event reports in a standardized format.

---

*A formulary is the list of pharmaceuticals that a health plan elects to cover as part of its contract with enrollees.

Chapter 12

Clinical Practice, Managed Care, and Health Insurance

In a 1997 *JAMA* study, 18.4 percent of adults who regularly took prescription medicines were concurrently taking at least one herbal medicine, a high-dose vitamin, or both.[1] The same study reported that only 15.1 percent of the people who said they used an herbal medicine in the past twelve months also saw an alternative practitioner. Without professional guidance from medical doctors or other practitioners, consumers may be inappropriately self-diagnosing and self-treating with botanicals and placing themselves at risk for drug-herb interactions.

EDUCATION OF MEDICAL PROFESSIONALS

The President's Commission identified a need for health care professionals to become more knowledgeable about herbal products. The educational system for medical doctors, pharmacists, nurse practitioners, physician assistants, and other medical professionals generally does not include training on herbal medicine. Training of allopathic professionals in botanical treatments therefore tends to be optional, uncoordinated, and unsupervised. The number of schools that include such training is slowly growing but is still not keeping abreast of consumer demand for professional guidance on herbal medicine.

Part of the resistance is due to a historic rift between herbal and allopathic medicine. Medical professionals are accustomed to single-compound pharmaceuticals and data from the gold standard randomized, placebo-controlled, double-blind human clinical trial study design. For reasons previously discussed, those types of data are rarely available for botanicals. Furthermore, practitioners of allopathic medicine are often uncomfortable with botanicals because these products are complex chemical mixtures rather than single compounds. Yet millions of consumers are using these products. Reports of adverse drug-herb interactions are increasing. Medical professionals have a responsibility to understand what is known so that they may better advise their patients on the appropriate use of botanicals. Not being informed can only exacerbate the problems.

COORDINATION OF TREATMENT

The lack of coordination of herbal treatments with concurrent allopathic care limits the overall quality of care. Many patients do not discuss the use of herbs with their physicians "because they believe that the physicians know little or nothing about these products and may be biased against them."[2] Many physicians dismiss such reports when they are provided. This situation raises at least two concerns. First, patients who self-medicate with botanicals may postpone needed medical attention. Their condition may have worsened by the time they do seek help. This problem arises with any form of self-medication. However, it is particularly pronounced when patients hesitate to disclose their use of botanicals to their physicians. Second, potential drug-herb interactions are more likely to be missed. Physicians have a small but growing body of research on this topic to turn to for guidance. The probability of these interactions occurring increases as consumer use of botanical products rises. The risk among the elderly is particularly acute because of the large number of pharmaceuticals they typically take.

Recently, data has begun to emerge on drug interactions with St. John's wort. It is thought that St. John's wort may induce the cytochrome P450 pathway, and hence the metabolism of many prescription drugs. Data are limited, but FDA issued a Public Health Advisory on February 10, 2000. It specifically advised against concurrent use of St. John's wort and indinavir and also warned of the possibility of a much broader risk involving other prescription drugs. The FDA urged health care professionals to ask their patients about use of St. John's wort products. St. John's wort is only the first botanical to receive attention regarding potential drug interactions and the importance of coordination with allopathic treatment. As botanicals are used more widely, the coordination issue grows ever more critical for the protection of public health.

It is certainly possible that allopathic treatments and herbal medicines together can broaden treatment options. When botanicals are considered, the overall outcome may be improved. For example, consider a patient who has chosen to stop taking pharmaceutical antidepressants because of side effects. This individual might be better off being treated with St. John's wort (as a monotherapy) rather than foregoing treatment altogether.

ACCESS TO BOTANICAL TREATMENT

Many people who could benefit from herbal medicines are not aware of these treatment options and/or cannot afford them. In part this problem stems from medical professionals being poorly informed about botanicals. Health insurance and managed care also play a role because they rarely cover professional consultations on herbal medicine or the products themselves. Even individuals who are aware of botanical treatment options may not be able to afford to pay out of pocket for them.

OPPORTUNITIES FOR COST SAVINGS

At a time when health care costs are a serious concern for the United States, the lower cost of botanical treatment alternatives may be increasingly relevant. Even for situations in which herbal medicines may cost less, be equally effective, and have fewer side effects than pharmaceuticals, these treatment options are not routinely presented to patients of allopathy.

There is an ongoing debate about whether nonallopathic treatments are being used as an adjunct to conventional therapies (i.e., are complementary) or as a substitute (i.e., alternative). The commonly used phrase *complementary and alternative medicine* captures these two possibilities. The economic impact of these two approaches are quite distinct. If patients are using botanicals in addition to conventional treatments, then overall expenditures may actually be higher. However, if an herbal medicine is used as a substitute, as in the case of St. John's wort or ginkgo, then cost savings could indeed be realized.

Chapter 13

Consumer Interests

CONSUMERS AS A POLITICAL FORCE

Since 1906, public opinion has often been the force that placed drug regulation on the national agenda. The Food, Drug and Cosmetic Act of 1938 (FDC Act) was enacted in response to the public outcry following the deaths from Elixir Sulfanilamide. The FDC Act was later amended to shift the burden of proof for safety and efficacy onto manufacturers—but only after the thalidomide tragedy of the early 1960s. Consumer opinion again played a major role in the legislative process that led to the Dietary Supplement Health and Education Act of 1994 (DSHEA). Much of the political force came from consumers demanding unrestricted access to botanicals. Since the amendment of the FDC Act with DSHEA, herbal medicines have grown to become a $5 billion market in the United States.

Looking at the regulatory history in the United States, a pattern seems to emerge. Consumers first demand ready access to medicinal products. A tragedy occurs. In response, consumers insist on tighter regulation. As David Kessler put it, "Americans view their government with a mixture of reliance and mistrust. We want to be free to choose whatever products we like until something goes wrong. Then we turn to our government and want to know why it happened and what the government is doing about it."[1] A widespread tragedy with botanicals has not yet occurred, and perhaps none will (although ephedra is getting close). However, if history repeats itself, as it often does, then it is only a matter of time before a disaster triggers tighter regulation of herbal medicines. Taking a less cynical view, proactive steps could be and are being taken to protect consumer interests as well as public health.

137

National opinion surveys suggest there is "broad public support for increased government regulation of these products . . . . a majority of Americans surveyed supported the following: to require that the Food and Drug Administration review the safety of new dietary supplements prior to their sale; to provide increased authority to remove from sale those products shown to be unsafe; and to increase government regulation to ensure that advertising claims about the health benefits of dietary supplements are true."[2] However, the same surveys report that consumers doubt the motivations of scientists and want the evidence on a product's dangers to be clear before the FDA considers removing it from the market.

SORTING THROUGH THE MORASS

From a public health standpoint, the situation with herbal medicines has two objectives to balance. On one hand, public safety is a concern. On the other hand, the public's health benefits from appropriate access to herbal medicines and information. Safety was discussed in Chapter 10, and access to herbal medicines and professional guidance was considered in Chapter 12. This chapter explores the issues surrounding consumer access to information and quality products.

Literature Quality Control and Access to Information

The literature on herbal medicines tends to be difficult to interpret, in part because of the widely disparate opinions and quality of data. Scientifically, this literature is complicated because it draws on several disciplines—e.g., botanical taxonomy, natural products chemistry, and pharmacology, to name a few. At best, the literature can only be as sound as the research that is funded. (The limitations of research funding for herbal medicines were discussed in Chapter 11.) Even the most experienced scientists find the literature challenging to interpret and often incomplete or of poor quality. Physicians and other medical professionals generally do not even read this literature. In the current regulatory environment, consumers are frequently taking it upon themselves to learn what they can. Consumers who use botanicals are usually self-medicating without professional guidance. Well-informed consumers try to understand the science, yet it is not realistic to expect laypeople to be able to interpret the complexities of this literature when even the most experienced professionals find it challenging and often ambiguous.

Most consumers do not read the scientific literature. Many rely on recommendations from family, friends, or health food store clerks. Many who take supplements (71 percent) indicate that they would continue using these products even if they were found to be ineffective in clinical trials.[3] Those who want to educate themselves on the science have access to a variety of information sources ranging widely in quality (e.g., infomercials, advertising, magazines, books, Web sites, and databases available on the Internet from research centers, nonprofit organizations, commercial enterprises, and the government). Section 5 of DSHEA allows stores to display third-party literature in a physically separate location from the dietary supplement products. These publications are exempt from labeling restrictions provided they convey a balanced view of the available scientific information and are not false or misleading.

The President's Commission encouraged manufacturers to use third-party literature "to help consumers use dietary supplements appropriately."[4] There are at least four problems with this approach. First, most consumers are not equipped to evaluate the scientific literature on their own. Second, even in the best cases the quality and quantity of the available literature is limited by the available data. Third, many of these publications do not cite the scientific, ethnobotanical, or ethnopharmacological literature, making the source of the information difficult to ascertain and evaluate. Fourth, this literature is not peer reviewed and is barely monitored at all. There is no official system in place for the FDA to monitor this literature.

Currently, medical professionals and consumers alike lack convenient systematic access to reliable, scientifically sound information on botanicals. This situation limits the quality of both self-care and supervised care. There are several projects under way that may improve access to information on botanicals. These projects include:

- The Office of Dietary Supplements (ODS) and the Food and Nutrition Information Center have collaborated to create a database called International Bibliographic Information on Dietary

Supplements (IBIDS). This resource is accessible through the ODS Web site.[5] It lists published, peer reviewed, international scientific literature on dietary supplements, including many botanicals.

- The ODS is also currently compiling information sheets on botanicals. These summaries will eventually be available over the Internet and hopefully will become a centralized source of high-quality information for consumers and professionals.
- A handbook of clinically tested botanicals on the U.S. market is now being written. It will distinguish products that have been clinically tested from those that contain purchased ingredients or ingredients that imitate a clinically tested product. Information in the book is being provided by the manufacturers. This book should help consumers and medical professionals begin to be able to identify the best herbal medicine products. Perhaps it will also provide an incentive for the botanicals industry to produce top quality, clinically tested products.

Substantiation of Structure/Function Label Claims

How to label botanicals was a highly contentious issue during the congressional debates that led to DSHEA. Many technical aspects were left unresolved, and DSHEA mandated the formation of the President's Commission on Dietary Supplement Labels to address these remaining issues.

Manufacturers are required by DSHEA to submit their structure/function claims to the FDA within the first thirty days of a product launch. However, the FDA estimated this reporting process would take only 0.5 to one hour per notification, and this estimate was not disputed by the industry. Clearly, a report that takes such a short time to prepare and submit can contain very limited information and provides little assurance that a product is safe as labeled.

DSHEA requires manufacturers to maintain substantiation files to back up their structure/function label claims, and the President's Commission suggested guidelines for the quality and type of information contained in these files. However, manufacturers are not required to make this documentation accessible to the FDA. Consequently, in practice, manufacturers set the quality standard for their own substantiation files with little or no monitoring.

Most of the scientific data in substantiation files are taken from publicly available sources because U.S. herbal medicine companies seldom conduct their own research (see Chapter 11 for more information). As a result, the data in even the best substantiation files are seldom product specific. Instead they tend to be based on the most closely related, publicly available information on the same plant species. The concern here is that the chemical composition of an herbal medicine product is not determined solely by the species from which it is made. A wide variety of products can be made from the same plant species. For example, if different parts of the plant and/or different chemical extraction processes are used, then the end products will differ in chemical composition. Differences in chemical composition, in turn, may well alter pharmacological activity. Because substantiation files rely heavily on publicly available information, the data they contain may or may not be relevant to the product in question.

Some manufacturers recognize the importance of self-monitoring in their industry. They also understand that if a tragedy results from the ingestion of an herbal product, a regulatory crackdown is likely to ensue. Some manufacturers are making concerted efforts to responsibly substantiate their label claims. However, in practice, companies have little power to monitor one another, and the quality (and presence) of substantiation files is essentially based on the honor principle, limited by the availability of relevant public information.

As discussed in Chapter 2, the controversy over appropriate wording for structure/function claims continues. Botanicals clearly do have biological action, as evidenced by the NIH-funded clinical trials and research centers. Yet because nearly all herbal medicines are legally classified as dietary supplements rather than drugs, label claims are restricted. Labels on botanical dietary supplement products are not permitted to indicate an intention to diagnose, treat, cure, mitigate, or prevent any disease. The semantics can be quite subtle when distinguishing between "maintaining normal function" (an acceptable dietary supplement claim) and "preventing or treating abnormal function" (which is potentially a disease claim).[6]

Unfortunately, these semantics do consumers a disservice. Rather than the labels providing clear information about the appropriate use of an herbal medicine, they give cryptic phrases. For many consumers these sanitized structure/function claims are simply euphemisms for what they gather from other sources to be the true indication. This situation does not promote the appropriate use of botanicals. In the absence of professional supervision, consumers need clear, direct labeling on botanicals. Structure/function claims have become an expensive game of semantics that contributes little to the improvement of public health. It is time for the U.S. regulatory debate on botanicals to move on to more meaningful topics.

Over-the-Counter Drug Status

DSHEA mandated the President's Commission to "evaluate how best to provide truthful, scientifically valid, and not misleading information to consumers so that such consumers may make informed and appropriate health care choices for themselves and their families."[7] In their report, the Commission commented that particular herbal products with therapeutic or preventive uses are recognized in other industrialized nations, and that in the United States these products are currently labeled with indirect statements about their uses. The Commission indicated that consumers would be better served if these herbal products were labeled with clear statements regarding therapeutic claims. The President's Commission strongly recommended that the "FDA promptly establish a review panel for OTC claims for botanical products that are proposed by manufacturers for drug uses"[8] and stated that the "FDA needs to give special attention to the feasibility of approving botanical remedies for OTC uses in cases in which sufficient evidence is available."[9] The President's Commission also advised that "more study is needed regarding the establishment of some alternative system for regulating botanical products that are used for purposes other than to supplement the diet but that cannot meet OTC drug requirements."[10] The Commission further noted the need for a comprehensive review of the approaches taken by other nations to regulating herbal medicinal products.

The FDA responded with an advance notice of proposed rule making in 1998 and its Guidance for Industry on botanical OTC drugs in 2000. The final rule is expected during 2002. As described in Chapter 2, by acknowledging the unique nature of botanicals and establishing new rules accordingly, this development represents a significant step in the right direction.

Continued progress on this front would be one of the most important changes in the current situation with herbal medicines in the United States. Creating a category for OTC botanicals would address many of the concerns raised in this analysis. Safety would be clearly demonstrated before marketing a product. Manufacturers would have an incentive to innovate, patent their products, and conduct research. Clinicians would be more comfortable recommending OTC products. Perhaps more health insurance plans, including Medicaid and Medicare, would cover botanicals, thereby increasing access to these less costly therapeutics. Consumers would have more access to medical supervision. Labels would provide clear, direct information on indications, dose, and potential side effects, eliminating the ambiguity of structure/function claims. Establishing a feasible approval process for approving botanical OTC products is a key step for the United States. It would simultaneously diminish the risk and augment the potential benefits from herbal medicines.

Chapter 14

The Roles of Business, Media, and the Government

THE ROLE OF BUSINESS AND MARKETING

The total number of herbal medicine products currently on the U.S. market is not known,[1] nor is the total number of plant species contained in these products known. Perhaps the best available estimate is from 1992 in *Herbs of Commerce*.[2] This book was published by the American Herbal Products Association, a trade organization representing the botanicals industry. It lists 550 plant species with 1,800 synonyms that are found in foods, dietary supplements, and medicinal products. Of course, individual species are frequently found in numerous products.

Sales estimates for herbal products tend to be rough because many of the distribution channels involved are outside the mainstream (e.g., health food stores, direct sales, multilevel marketing). While the specific figures vary, the trends are fairly apparent: Sales rose sharply after 1995, peaked in 1998 or 1999, leveled off in 2000, and began to decline in 2001, with sales of St. John's wort and ginkgo falling the most.[3,4,5,6] In 2001, the twenty top-selling botanicals comprising 62 percent of sales in natural food stores surveyed in the United States were: echinacea, garlic, ginkgo, saw palmetto, ginseng, grape seed extract, green tea, St. John's wort, bilberry, aloe, cranberry, milk thistle, ginger, olive leaf extract, ma huang and other ephedra products, dong quai, black cohosh, astragalus, siberian ginseng, and psyllium.[7] Of note, echinacea has consistently led sales since 1995 but has not yet been the subject of an NIH-funded clinical trial.

Private businesses are playing a powerful role in the situation with herbal medicines. In many ways, consumers of botanicals are at the mercy of the manufacturers. The paucity of research can be traced to the reluctance of manufacturers to conduct studies. In turn, their reluctance can be explained by the fact that they are not innovating and patenting their products. If research efforts are going to expand significantly beyond the NIH's efforts, manufacturers will need to contribute most of the funding.

Producers of herbal medicines are enjoying substantial cost savings because their products do not require premarket approval from the FDA. This creates a somewhat unlevel playing field with pharmaceuticals (although much of the economic advantage of dietary supplements is lost because they are for the most part unpatentable). Furthermore, in contrast to other countries where botanicals are regulated as drugs, no registration fees are required in the United States. In return, manufacturers have a responsibility to self-monitor their own firms as well as the industry at large. It is in the best interests of manufacturers to work with the FDA to establish good manufacturing practices as quickly as possible. Quality control throughout the supply chain is critical, as demonstrated by the adulteration case described in Chapter 9. Manufacturers have a responsibility to maintain the highest quality substantiation files possible. Once their products are marketed, if adverse events are reported to them, they have an ethical obligation to voluntarily submit as complete a report as possible to the FDA. In their marketing, they should be cautious about the information they give consumers and avoid generating misleading advertising. All of these expectations amount to a need for high ethical standards in a profit-driven environment. It is dubious to what extent the industry as a whole can maintain such a level of self-compliance. Falling short on any one of these points represents a significant risk to public health. It is a delicate situation. One tragedy could tip the balance and trigger much tighter regulations that would redefine this industry. In the meantime, as the marketplace consolidates, companies are beginning to choose between targeting high-end niches with clinically tested products and low-end markets with commodity-like products.[8]

THE ROLE OF MEDIA

Because consumers are mainly self-medicating with botanicals, the popular press becomes a particularly significant influence on consumer behavior. Magazines such as *Reader's Digest* and *Prevention* and newspaper columns such as Jane Brody's "Personal Health" column in *The New York Times* frequently feature herbal medicines. Several problems arise when these publications become a key source of information for consumers. Although the authors may be better informed than the average consumer, they are journalists, not scientists or medical professionals. As journalists, they need to sell newspapers and magazines, and they may sensationalize information toward that end. Their ability to interpret scientific studies is limited and the information they provide is frequently not cited. These publications are not peer reviewed and are barely monitored by the FDA or the scientific or medical communities.

For example, in 1997 after the meta-analysis of St. John's wort for mild depression was published in the *British Medical Journal,*[9] *The New York Times* ran columns two days in a row on this topic.[10,11] Most of the information was reported accurately, although the statements it made were poorly cited. Some errors were made, such as indicating that the meta-analysis included twenty-eight studies when in fact it included only twenty-three. However, the greatest problem was the sensationalism. The first column was titled "In Germany, Humble Herb Is Rival to Prozac." The article pointed out that in Germany St. John's wort products outsell Prozac by four to one. This statement is problematic because it was based on sales figures, not on clinical trials or observational studies. No clinical trial or epidemiological study has specifically compared St. John's wort and Prozac. In an article that consumers read for its lay interpretation of the scientific literature, such an insinuation is misleading.

THE ROLE OF THE FEDERAL GOVERNMENT

The primary responsibility of the federal government with herbal medicines is to protect and promote public health. This section evaluates the impact of surveillance, funding, and federal regulations.

Surveillance

For herbal medicines, surveillance is passive and tends to yield poor quality data on adverse events. Because the vast majority of botanicals are safe, the surveillance system for herbal medicines should be designed accordingly. Its priority should be to quickly zero in on the rare botanical that is hazardous. The current passive surveillance system for herbal medicines is inadequate by any standard, but it is particularly lacking in light of the absence of premarket approval for these products.

Epidemiological research, as discussed in Chapter 11, would greatly augment surveillance.

Funding

NIH research funding for botanicals has increased dramatically in recent years. Hopefully, this signals a new era of support for herbal medicine research.

DSHEA mandated the establishment of the NIH Office of Dietary Supplements (ODS) and authorized a $5 million budget for 1994. However, Congress appropriated only $1 million and the ODS director funded the start-up costs through the NIH Director's Discretionary Fund. Beginning in 1996, the ODS budget has been a line item in the Office of the Director's budget. In 1996 and 1997 the ODS budget was still only $1 million. In 1997, the President's Commission report recommended that the ODS be funded with the full $5 million authorized by DSHEA. In 1998, the budget grew to $1.5 million and in 1999 to $3.5 million. The limitations on the ODS appropriations constrained what it could contribute. During these initial five years, consumers were sorely in need of a reliable information source and other government agencies could have benefited from sound advice on dietary supplements. ODS was well positioned to provide those services but underfunding limited the extent of its activities.

Federal Regulations

Herbal medicines throughout the world, including the United States, are usually consumed for their putative pharmacological effects, however subtle. Rarely are herbal medicines taken for their nutritional content. Classifying botanicals as dietary supplements is not in line with their generally intended use; it is a case of forcing a square peg into a round hole. Not surprisingly, the regulation of botanical dietary supplements has been fraught with difficulties. Unfortunately, the primary goal of protecting and promoting public health has often suffered in the process.

Many of the shortcomings of DSHEA have been elucidated in previous chapters. The absence of a reasonable premarket approval process for botanicals, either as dietary supplements or as over-the-counter drugs, has allowed the marketplace to become awash in products of widely varying quality. As a result, the public's health is at considerable risk. Passive surveillance systems have constrained the government's postmarket protection of public health. Labeling restrictions on structure/function claims prevent consumers from being clearly and directly informed about the intended use of herbal medicine products. Consequently, consumers and medical professionals lack the information they need to use these products to promote health. Implementing the labeling requirements for the nutritional content of botanicals has been time consuming and expensive for government and manufacturers and has provided little meaningful information for consumers of botanicals. These problems place public health at risk and severely limit the potential benefits consumers can derive from using herbal medicines.

Classifying botanicals as dietary supplements is limiting their contribution to public health. Classifying botanicals in the same way that pharmaceutical drugs are classified may not be much better. The pharmaceutical drug approval process is designed for patented, single molecular entities. Herbal medicines are generally not patentable and are usually complex chemical mixtures with several active constituents. They also have a long history of use, which is worthy of consideration. Public health would best be served if herbal medicines were classified and approved under a separate process specifically designed for their unique safety and efficacy issues. Fortunately, the new FDA policies on botanical drugs appear to be headed in this direction.

Regarding safety, many botanicals have a long history of safe use. This evidence should be considered in the evaluation of safety and, where appropriate, used to accelerate the approval process. The Canadian system of dividing botanicals according to the risk associated with them is a rational and useful model. It acknowledges that many botanicals are quite safe while others carry considerable risk. Such an approach allows attention to be focused on a small number of higher-risk botanicals without blocking safe products from reaching the market quickly. The higher-risk botanicals should require premarket approval based on product-specific human safety data.

Regarding efficacy, several major changes are needed.

- Currently the NIH is funding the most substantive clinical research on herbal medicines in the United States. However, the federal government should not be expected to fund all of the research while manufacturers fund very little or none.
- Efficacy needs to be addressed directly. Structure/function claims serve only to blur information and create ambiguity. NIH is now funding clinical studies and research centers on the "biological effects" of botanicals. The regulations need to be updated to reflect an equally straightforward approach to efficacy. The new rules for OTC botanicals may help. Meanwhile, in the absence of a clear path, an ad hoc procedure is emerging: a small trial is conducted and its results are then published in a major medical journal, which then leads to an NIH trial. However, this approach will be feasible only for a handful of leading edge products due to the expense involved.
- U.S. monographs on botanicals (as part of *The United States Pharmacopoeia*) should be established to clearly delineate the efficacy (among other properties) of these products. The German Commission E monographs provide one model for this approach. Once monograph standards are established, then manufacturers could be required to adhere to a monograph to make the specific efficacy claims it contains. This approach would help bring standardization to U.S. products and streamline the FDA's monitoring. The proposed regulations for OTC botanicals would allow manufacturers to seek OTC monograph status for their products. However, such status would confer no exclusivity. It therefore remains unclear whether competing manufacturers would be willing and able to successfully develop OTC monographs at their own expense. Under the proposed rule, it is also uncertain how these monographs would be standardized for optimal quality, safety, and efficacy since multiple firms could submit applications for similar products.
- For the purpose of monographs, historical (traditional) use should be considered even if the data are largely from foreign

countries. With such limited resources available to sort out the situation with botanicals, there is little reason to duplicate existing information. Both traditional use and published scientific data should be evaluated to validate the plant species for the particular therapeutic use designated in the monograph. For lower-risk species, traditional-use data alone may be sufficient. For intermediate- and higher-risk species, additional scientific data are needed to clarify the risk-benefit rato. The FDA's final rule of January 23, 2002, provides a procedure for including foreign experience on a time and extent application. However, it remains to be seen whether these requirements are achievable or turn out to be too cumbersome to be practical.

- For products that do not comply with a monograph, the manufacturer should have the option of continuing to market the product as is (a dietary supplement), or seeking product-specific OTC botanical status through a new drug application. In either case, label claims should be based on *product-specific* data. Under DSHEA, borrowing science from other products that may or may not be relevant has become commonplace and has created unintelligible scientific ambiguity in label claims. If product-specific data become a legal requirement, then even without a patent manufacturers would be able to justify the expense of research since the resulting data would be of no value to their competitors. This one change has the potential to dramatically increase the quantity and quality of research conducted in the United States on herbal medicines. It could also drastically improve the reliability of label information. In a positive development along these lines, the FDA's proposed OTC botanical rules would provide exclusivity both for products that lack patents (three years) and for those with patent protection (five years).

- For the vast majority of products that present no particular cause for safety concerns, clinical intervention trials could be conducted postmarket to clarify efficacy. The products would not even need to be taken off the market. Manufacturers could use ongoing sales to fund their research. Considering the millions of Americans who are already taking botanicals, manufacturers should be able to gather data from large, high-quality human studies. Conducting such research would likely be a boon for marketing, especially if manufacturers offer free product to participants. The regulations could require these studies to be completed within a specific time frame.

- Postmarket epidemiological studies should be required for herbal medicine products and especially higher-risk products and those taken to treat chronic diseases. Study designs should allow detection of both acute and chronic toxicity, as well as therapeutic benefits. Manufacturers should fund these studies, but many possibilities exist for collaboration. Because millions of Americans are already using herbal medicines, large sample sizes should be quite obtainable. Such data would augment the current passive surveillance system.

- Government-funded research needs to continue to focus on therapeutic areas of greatest public health importance where existing data suggest herbal medicines may be able to offer improvements to existing treatment options. St. John's wort for depression and ginkgo for Alzheimer's disease are appropriate choices. Echinacea for immune system support would be a prime candidate for future studies.

- Government-funded research should include a cost effectiveness arm so that comparisons can be made based on data from the same clinical trials.

An approval system with these features would go a long way toward addressing many of the public health concerns raised in this book. This process could be imposed retroactively, similar to the way the OTC monograph system sorted through products that were already on the market to bring them into compliance with new safety and efficacy requirements. Ideally, these changes could be made proactively, putting an updated botanical approval process in place before a public health tragedy, such as thalidomide, occurs. With this revised system, the government would benefit from a more straightforward process, manufacturers would have new opportunities to profit from innovation and research, and consumers would enjoy higher-quality products and the associated health improvements.

PART V:
CONCLUSION

Chapter 15

Summary and Recommendations

SUMMARY OF FINDINGS

In general, in the United States herbal medicines are used by laypeople to self-medicate their self-diagnosed maladies. Most consumers believe these medicines are safe because they are natural and sold over the counter without a prescription. The regulatory climate under the Dietary Supplement Health and Education Act of 1994 has allowed a rapid proliferation of botanical products in the U.S. market. Because herbal medicines are pharmacologically active, the concurrent increase in use and product proliferation raises a number of public health concerns:

- *Coordination of treatment.* Coordination with concurrent allopathic care is poor, which limits the overall quality of care. Consumers may be inappropriately self-diagnosing and self-treating with botanicals without guidance from professionals. The probability of overlooking potential drug-herb interactions increases as more consumers use botanical products.
- *Access to botanical treatment.* Health insurance and managed care rarely cover professional consultation for herbal medicines or the products themselves. Consequently, many people who could benefit are not aware of botanical treatment options. Even those who are aware of botanical options may not be able to afford to pay out of pocket for them.
- *Opportunities for cost savings.* At a time when health care costs are a serious concern for the United States, the lower cost of botanical treatment alternatives may be increasingly relevant. Even in situations where herbal medicines may cost less, be equally effective, or have fewer side effects than pharmaceuticals, these

treatment options are not routinely presented to patients of allopathy in the United States.

- *Product quality control.* Botanical product quality control standards vary widely and are difficult for both consumers and professionals to assess. Even the best informed consumers and professionals struggle to distinguish among quality, mediocre, and dangerous products and/or doses.
- *Safety.* Postmarket surveillance of adverse events is passive. Numerous points exist in the supply chain at which safety may be a concern. Drug-botanical interactions are being reported more frequently.
- *Structure/function claims.* These label claims on botanical dietary supplements create ambiguity and prevent consumers from being clearly and directly informed about the intended use of herbal medicinal products.
- *Literature quality control.* Too many reference books and articles on herbal medicine do not cite the scientific, ethnobotanical, or ethnopharmacological literature, making the sources of the information difficult to ascertain and evaluate.
- *Access to information.* Physicians and consumers alike lack convenient systematic access to reliable, scientifically sound information on botanicals. The current system is suboptimal for both self-care and supervised care.
- *Education.* The education system for medical doctors and pharmacists generally does not include training on herbal medicine. Training of allopathic professionals in botanical treatments therefore tends to be optional, uncoordinated, and unsupervised. The potential for drug-botanical interactions is likely to be overlooked.
- *Research.* Research funding for clinical trials on herbal medicine is very limited in the United States. As a result, most of the available data come from other countries and until January 2002 were not applicable under U.S. law. A public health perspective can contribute to establishing meaningful funding priorities.
- *Clinical studies on specific products.* Although millions of Americans are consuming herbal medicines, very few of these products have undergone rigorous preclinical or clinical trials to optimize product standardization, dosage, formulation, and treatment regimens.

- *Patent protection.* Because of the difficulties with patent protection of botanicals, few incentives exist for manufacturers to contribute to research funding or to conduct research of their own. The proposed FDA rule on OTC botanicals may improve incentives by allowing exclusivity for unpatented products.
- *Epidemiological data.* Surveillance systems are currently focused on adverse reactions. There is a notable absence of coordinated effort to gather quality epidemiological data to monitor and systematically evaluate the *positive* effects of botanicals. The potential power of such a data set would be particularly significant for some of the most commonly used botanicals that are consumed by millions of Americans.
- *Need for a modified approval system.* Botanicals differ sufficiently from foods, nutritional supplements, and drugs to warrant a modified approval system. The FDA's proposed rule on OTC botanicals acknowledged this distinction for the first time in United States history. The FDA's final rule of January 2002 allowing foreign experience to be considered in time and extent applications and its proposed rule on OTC botanicals are major steps in the right direction.

RECOMMENDATIONS

The U.S. situation with botanicals is highly complex. There are no simple or quick solutions. The following recommendations are intended to address the core public health issues and hopefully stimulate discussion in fruitful directions. The approach outlined could move the United States a long way toward cleaning up the botanicals marketplace. Bear in mind that existing products need not be removed from the market for these recommendations to be implemented. Yet motivated manufacturers could begin to better differentiate their products by gaining access to and complying with optional new approval procedures.

1. Form an expert panel on botanicals and clearly define its mandate and authority.
2. Categorize products by risk, and label and regulate accordingly.
   - Especially for higher-risk products and those taken to treat chronic diseases, require rigorous postmarket observational

studies paid for by the manufacturer and monitored by a third party. Design these studies to elucidate safety (with acute and chronic use), efficacy, and cost-effectiveness.

- For lower-risk products, compile monographs based on historical data if these data are all that is available. Allow specific disease claims for products that comply with these monographs.
- For intermediate- and higher-risk products, compile monographs (as part of *The United States Pharmacopoeia*) based on historical (traditional) use and scientific data. Allow only those products that comply with the monographs to be labeled with the disease claims specified in the monographs. This approach would provide an incentive for manufacturers to follow the monographs. With proper labeling, consumers could then readily identify whether a product is monograph compliant or not.

3. Compile standard monographs on the most widely used botanicals first. Monographs on the twenty-five most common plant species would cover a large portion (perhaps 70 percent) of the botanicals marketplace. Monographs should cover (but not be limited to):
   - Botanical quality control requirements and references
   - Good manufacturing practices and quality control requirements
   - Permitted disease claims
   - Foreign and historical use data so as not to duplicate studies unnecessarily

4. Establish an over-the-counter drug approval process specifically for botanicals that encourages innovation beyond standard monographs. Adapt approval procedures for botanicals to include consideration of traditional use, foreign data, and other scientific evidence.

5. For botanicals that do not comply with a monograph, require product-specific data for OTC botanicals so that patenting becomes less relevant and manufacturers have an incentive to fund and/or conduct premarket and postmarket research.

6. Encourage education of health care professionals on botanicals and potential drug-herb interactions.

To a large extent, the U.S. situation with botanicals has been and will probably continue to be consumer driven. The recommendations provided here are intended to promote a marketplace in which consumers will enjoy both greater health benefits from botanicals and improved protection from risk.

Appendix A

U.S. Dietary Supplement Health and Education Act of 1994

Public Law 103-417—October 25, 1994
"Dietary Supplement Health and Education Act"
S.784
One Hundred Third Congress of the United States of America
AT THE SECOND SESSION
Begun and held at the City of Washington
on Tuesday, the twenty-fifth day of January,
one thousand nine hundred and ninety-four
An Act
To amend the Federal Food, Drug, and Cosmetic Act to establish
standards with respect to dietary supplements, and for other purposes.
Be it enacted by the Senate and House of Representatives
of the United States of America in Congress assembled,

SECTION 1. SHORT TITLE; REFERENCE; TABLE OF CONTENTS.

(a) SHORT TITLE.—This Act may be cited as the "Dietary Supplement Health and Education Act of 1994".

(b) REFERENCE.—Whenever in this Act an amendment or repeal is expressed in terms of an amendment to, or repeal of, a section or other provision, the reference shall be considered to be made to a section or other provision of the Federal Food, Drug, and Cosmetic Act.

(c) TABLE OF CONTENTS.—The table of contents of this Act is as follows:

Sec. 6. Statements of nutritional support.
Sec. 7. Dietary supplement ingredient labeling and nutrition information labeling.
Sec. 8. New dietary ingredients.
Sec. 9. Good manufacturing practices.
Sec. 10. Conforming amendments.
Sec. 11. Withdrawal of the regulations and notice.
Sec. 12. Commission on dietary supplement labels.
Sec. 13. Office of dietary supplements.

SEC. 2. FINDINGS.

Congress finds that—

(1) improving the health status of United States citizens ranks at the top of the national priorities of the Federal Government;

(2) the importance of nutrition and the benefits of dietary supplements to health promotion and disease prevention have been documented increasingly in scientific studies;

(3)(A) there is a link between the ingestion of certain nutrients or dietary supplements and the prevention of chronic diseases such as cancer, heart disease, and osteoporosis; and

(B) clinical research has shown that several chronic diseases can be prevented simply with a healthful diet, such as a diet that is low in fat, saturated fat, cholesterol, and sodium, with a high proportion of plant-based foods;

(4) healthful diets may mitigate the need for expensive medical procedures, such as coronary bypass surgery or angioplasty;

(5) preventive health measures, including education, good nutrition, and appropriate use of safe nutritional supplements will limit the incidence of chronic diseases, and reduce long-term health care expenditures;

(6)(A) promotion of good health and healthy lifestyles improves and extends lives while reducing health care expenditures; and

(B) reduction in health care expenditures is of paramount importance to the future of the country and the economic well-being of the country;

(7) there is a growing need for emphasis on the dissemination of information linking nutrition and long-term good health;

(8) consumers should be empowered to make choices about preventive health care programs based on data from scientific studies of health benefits related to particular dietary supplements;

(9) national surveys have revealed that almost 50 percent of the 260,000,000 Americans regularly consume dietary supplements of vitamins, minerals, or herbs as a means of improving their nutrition;

(10) studies indicate that consumers are placing increased reliance on the use of nontraditional health care providers to avoid the excessive costs of traditional medical services and to obtain more holistic consideration of their needs;

(11) the United States will spend over $1,000,000,000,000 on health care in 1994, which is about 12 percent of the Gross National Product of the United States, and this amount and percentage will continue to increase unless significant efforts are undertaken to reverse the increase;

(12)(A) the nutritional supplement industry is an integral part of the economy of the United States;

(B) the industry consistently projects a positive trade balance; and

(C) the estimated 600 dietary supplement manufacturers in the United States produce approximately 4,000 products, with total annual sales of such products alone reaching at least $4,000,000,000;

(13) although the Federal Government should take swift action against products that are unsafe or adulterated, the Federal Government should not take any actions to impose unreasonable regulatory barriers limiting or slowing the flow of safe products and accurate information to consumers;

(14) dietary supplements are safe within a broad range of intake, and safety problems with the supplements are relatively rare; and

(15)(A) legislative action that protects the right of access of consumers to safe dietary supplements is necessary in order to promote wellness; and

(B) a rational Federal framework must be established to supersede the current ad hoc, patchwork regulatory policy on dietary supplements.

SEC. 3. DEFINITIONS.

(a) DEFINITION OF CERTAIN FOODS AS DIETARY SUPPLEMENTS.—Section 201 (21 U.S.C. 321) is amended by adding at the end the following:

"(ff) The term 'dietary supplement'—

"(1) means a product (other than tobacco) intended to supplement the diet that bears or contains one or more of the following dietary ingredients:

"(A) a vitamin;

"(B) a mineral;

"(C) an herb or other botanical;

"(D) an amino acid;

"(E) a dietary substance for use by man to supplement the diet by increasing the total dietary intake; or

"(F) a concentrate, metabolite, constituent, extract, or combination of any ingredient described in clause (A), (B), (C), (D), or (E);

"(2) means a product that—

"(A)(i) is intended for ingestion in a form described in section 411(c)(1)(B)(i); or

"(ii) complies with section 411(c)(1)(B)(ii);

"(B) is not represented for use as a conventional food or as a sole item of a meal or the diet; and

"(C) is labeled as a dietary supplement; and

"(3) does—

"(A) include an article that is approved as a new drug under section 505, certified as an antibiotic under section 507, or licensed as a biologic under section 351 of the Public Health Service Act (42 U.S.C. 262) and was, prior to such approval, certification, or license, marketed as a dietary supplement or as a food unless the Secretary has issued a regulation, after notice and comment, finding that the article, when used as or in a dietary supplement under the conditions of use and dosages set forth in the labeling for such dietary supplement, is unlawful under section 402(f); and

"(B) not include—

"(i) an article that is approved as a new drug under section 505, certified as an antibiotic under section 507, or licensed as a biologic under section 351 of the Public Health Service Act (42 U.S.C. 262), or

"(ii) an article authorized for investigation as a new drug, antibiotic, or biological for which substantial clinical investigations have been instituted and for which the existence of such investigations has been made public,

which was not before such approval, certification, licensing, or authorization marketed as a dietary supplement or as a food unless the Secretary, in the Secretary's discretion, has issued a regulation, after notice and comment, finding that the article would be lawful under this Act.

Except for purposes of section 201(g), a dietary supplement shall be deemed to be a food within the meaning of this Act.".

(b) EXCLUSION FROM DEFINITION OF FOOD ADDITIVE.—Section 201(s) (21 U.S.C. 321(s)) is amended—

(1) by striking "or" at the end of subparagraph (4);

(2) by striking the period at the end of subparagraph (5) and inserting "; or"; and

(3) by adding at the end the following new subparagraph: "(6) an ingredient described in paragraph (ff) in, or intended for use in, a dietary supplement.".

(c) FORM OF INGESTION.—Section 411(c)(1)(B) (21 U.S.C. 350(c)(1)(B)) is amended—

(1) in clause (i), by inserting "powder, softgel, gelcap," after "capsule,"; and

(2) in clause (ii), by striking "does not simulate and".

SEC. 4. SAFETY OF DIETARY SUPPLEMENTS AND BURDEN OF PROOF ON FDA.

Section 402 (21 U.S.C. 342) is amended by adding at the end the following:

"(f)(1) If it is a dietary supplement or contains a dietary ingredient that—

"(A) presents a significant or unreasonable risk of illness or injury under—

"(i) conditions of use recommended or suggested in labeling, or

"(ii) if no conditions of use are suggested or recommended in the labeling, under ordinary conditions of use;

"(B) is a new dietary ingredient for which there is inadequate information to provide reasonable assurance that such ingredient does not present a significant or unreasonable risk of illness or injury;

"(C) the Secretary declares to pose an imminent hazard to public health or safety, except that the authority to make such declaration shall not be delegated and the Secretary shall promptly after such a declaration initiate a proceeding in accordance with sections 554 and 556 of title 5, United States Code, to affirm or withdraw the declaration; or

"(D) is or contains a dietary ingredient that renders it adulterated under paragraph (a)(1) under the conditions of use recommended or suggested in the labeling of such dietary supplement.

In any proceeding under this subparagraph, the United States shall bear the burden of proof on each element to show that a dietary supplement is adulterated. The court shall decide any issue under this paragraph on a de novo basis.

"(2) Before the Secretary may report to a United States attorney a violation of paragraph (1)(A) for a civil proceeding, the person against whom such proceeding would be initiated shall be given appropriate notice and the opportunity to present views, orally and in writing, at least ten days before such notice, with regard to such proceeding.".

SEC. 5. DIETARY SUPPLEMENT CLAIMS.

Chapter IV (21 U.S.C. 341 et seq.) is amended by inserting after section 403A the following new section:

"DIETARY SUPPLEMENT LABELING EXEMPTIONS

"SEC. 403B. (a) IN GENERAL.—A publication, including an article, a chapter in a book, or an official abstract of a peer-reviewed scientific publication that appears in an article and was prepared by the author or the editors of the publication, which is reprinted in its entirety, shall not be defined as labeling when used in connection with the sale of a dietary supplement to consumers when it—

"(1) is not false or misleading;

"(2) does not promote a particular manufacturer or brand of a dietary supplement;

"(3) is displayed or presented, or is displayed or presented with other such items on the same subject matter, so as to present a balanced view of the available scientific information on a dietary supplement;

"(4) if displayed in an establishment, is physically separate from the dietary supplements; and

"(5) does not have appended to it any information by sticker or any other method.

"(b) APPLICATION.—Subsection (a) shall not apply to or restrict a retailer or wholesaler of dietary supplements in any way whatsoever in the sale of books or other publications as a part of the business of such retailer or wholesaler.

"(c) BURDEN OF PROOF.—In any proceeding brought under subsection (a), the burden of proof shall be on the United States to establish that an article or other such matter is false or misleading.".

SEC. 6. STATEMENTS OF NUTRITIONAL SUPPORT.

Section 403(r) (21 U.S.C. 343(r)) is amended by adding at the end the following:

"(6) For purposes of paragraph (r)(1)(B), a statement for a dietary supplement may be made if—

"(A) the statement claims a benefit related to a classical nutrient deficiency disease and discloses the prevalence of such disease in the

United States, describes the role of a nutrient or dietary ingredient intended to affect the structure or function in humans, characterizes the documented mechanism by which a nutrient or dietary ingredient acts to maintain such structure or function, or describes general well-being from consumption of a nutrient or dietary ingredient,

"(B) the manufacturer of the dietary supplement has substantiation that such statement is truthful and not misleading, and

"(C) the statement contains, prominently displayed and in boldface type, the following: 'This statement has not been evaluated by the Food and Drug Administration. This product is not intended to diagnose, treat, cure, or prevent any disease.'.

A statement under this subparagraph may not claim to diagnose, mitigate, treat, cure, or prevent a specific disease or class of diseases. If the manufacturer of a dietary supplement proposes to make a statement described in the first sentence of this subparagraph in the labeling of the dietary supplement, the manufacturer shall notify the Secretary no later than 30 days after the first marketing of the dietary supplement with such statement that such a statement is being made.".

SEC. 7. DIETARY SUPPLEMENT INGREDIENT LABELING AND NUTRITION INFORMATION LABELING.

(a) MISBRANDED SUPPLEMENTS.—Section 403 (21 U.S.C. 343) is amended by adding at the end the following:

"(s) If—

"(1) it is a dietary supplement; and

"(2) (A) the label or labeling of the supplement fails to list—

"(i) the name of each ingredient of the supplement that is described in section 201(ff); and

"(ii)(I) the quantity of each such ingredient; or

"(II) with respect to a proprietary blend of such ingredients, the total quantity of all ingredients in the blend;

"(B) the label or labeling of the dietary supplement fails to identify the product by using the term 'dietary supplement', which term may be modified with the name of such an ingredient;

"(C) the supplement contains an ingredient described in section 201(ff)(1)(C), and the label or labeling of the supplement fails to identify any part of the plant from which the ingredient is derived;

"(D) the supplement—

"(i) is covered by the specifications of an official compendium;

"(ii) is represented as conforming to the specifications of an official compendium; and

"(iii) fails to so conform; or

"(E) the supplement—

"(i) is not covered by the specifications of an official compendium; and

"(ii)(I) fails to have the identity and strength that the supplement is represented to have; or

"(II) fails to meet the quality (including tablet or capsule disintegration), purity, or compositional specifications, based on validated assay or other appropriate methods, that the supplement is represented to meet.".

(b) SUPPLEMENT LISTING ON NUTRITION LABELING.—Section 403(q)(5)(F) (21 U.S.C. 343(q)(5)(F)) is amended to read as follows:

"(F) A dietary supplement product (including a food to which section 411 applies) shall comply with the requirements of subparagraphs (1) and (2) in a manner which is appropriate for the product and which is specified in regulations of the Secretary which shall provide that—

"(i) nutrition information shall first list those dietary ingredients that are present in the product in a significant amount and for which a recommendation for daily consumption has been established by the Secretary, except that a dietary ingredient shall not be required to be listed if it is not present in a significant amount, and shall list any other dietary ingredient present and identified as having no such recommendation;

"(ii) the listing of dietary ingredients shall include the quantity of each such ingredient (or of a proprietary blend of such ingredients) per serving;

"(iii) the listing of dietary ingredients may include the source of a dietary ingredient; and

"(iv) the nutrition information shall immediately precede the ingredient information required under subclause (i), except that no ingredient identified pursuant to subclause (i) shall be required to be identified a second time.".

(c) PERCENTAGE LEVEL CLAIMS.—Section 403(r)(2) (21 U.S.C. 343(r)(2)) is amended by adding after clause (E) the following:

"(F) Subclause (i) clause (A) does not apply to a statement in the labeling of a dietary supplement that characterizes the percentage level of a dietary ingredient for which the Secretary has not established a reference daily intake, daily recommended value, or other recommendation for daily consumption.".

(d) VITAMINS AND MINERALS.—Section 411(b)(2) (21 U.S.C. 350(b)(2)) is amended—

(1) by striking "vitamins or minerals" and inserting "dietary supplement ingredients described in section 201(ff)";

(2) by striking "(2)(A)" and inserting "(2)"; and

(3) by striking subparagraph (B).

(e) EFFECTIVE DATE.—Dietary supplements—

(1) may be labeled after the date of the enactment of this Act in accordance with the amendments made by this section, and

(2) shall be labeled after December 31, 1996, in accordance with such amendments.

SEC. 8. NEW DIETARY INGREDIENTS.

Chapter IV of the Federal Food, Drug, and Cosmetic Act is amended by adding at the end the following:

"NEW DIETARY INGREDIENTS

"SEC. 413. (a) IN GENERAL—A dietary supplement which contains a new dietary ingredient shall be deemed adulterated under section 402(f) unless it meets one of the following requirements:

"(1) The dietary supplement contains only dietary ingredients which have been present in the food supply as an article used for food in a form in which the food has not been chemically altered.

"(2) There is a history of use or other evidence of safety establishing that the dietary ingredient when used under the conditions recommended or suggested in the labeling of the dietary supplement will reasonably be expected to be safe and, at least 75 days before being introduced or delivered for introduction into interstate commerce, the manufacturer or distributor of the dietary ingredient or dietary supplement provides the Secretary with information, including any citation to published articles, which is the basis on which the manufacturer or distributor has concluded that a dietary supplement containing such dietary ingredient will reasonably be expected to be safe.

The Secretary shall keep confidential any information provided under paragraph (2) for 90 days following its receipt. After the expiration of such 90 days, the Secretary shall place such information on public display, except matters in the information which are trade secrets or otherwise confidential, commercial information.

"(b) PETITION.—Any person may file with the Secretary a petition proposing the issuance of an order prescribing the conditions under which a new dietary ingredient under its intended conditions of use will reasonably be expected to be safe. The Secretary shall make a decision on such petition within 180 days of the date the petition is filed with the Secretary. For purposes of chapter 7 of title 5, United States Code, the decision of the Secretary shall be considered final agency action.

"(c) DEFINITION.—For purposes of this section, the term 'new dietary ingredient' means a dietary ingredient that was not marketed in the United States before October 15, 1994 and does not include any dietary ingredient which was marketed in the United States before October 15, 1994.".

SEC. 9. GOOD MANUFACTURING PRACTICES.

Section 402 (21 U.S.C. 342), as amended by section 4, is amended by adding at the end the following:

"(g)(1) If it is a dietary supplement and it has been prepared, packed, or held under conditions that do not meet current good manufacturing practice regulations, including regulations requiring, when necessary, expiration date labeling, issued by the Secretary under subparagraph (2).

"(2) The Secretary may by regulation prescribe good manufacturing practices for dietary supplements. Such regulations shall be modeled after current good manufacturing practice regulations for food and may not impose standards for which there is no current and generally available analytical methodology. No standard of current good manufacturing practice may be imposed unless such standard is included in a regulation promulgated after notice and opportunity for comment in accordance with chapter 5 of title 5, United States Code.".

SEC. 10. CONFORMING AMENDMENTS.

(a) SECTION 201.—The last sentence of section 201(g)(1) (21 U.S.C. 321(g)(1)) is amended to read as follows: 'A food or dietary supplement for which a claim, subject to sections 403(r)(1)(B) and 403(r)(3) or sections 403(r)(1)(B) and 403(r)(5)(D), is made in accordance with the requirements of section 403(r) is not a drug solely because the label or the labeling contains such a claim. A food, dietary ingredient, or dietary supplement for which a truthful and not misleading statement is made in accordance with section 403(r)(6) is not a drug under clause (C) solely because the label or the labeling contains such a statement.".

(b) SECTION 301.—Section 301 (21 U.S.C. 331) is amended by adding at the end the following:

"(u) The introduction or delivery for introduction into interstate commerce of a dietary supplement that is unsafe under section 413.".

(c) SECTION 403.—Section 403 (21 U.S.C. 343), as amended by section 7, is amended by adding after paragraph (s) the following: "A dietary supplement shall not be deemed misbranded solely because its label or labeling contains directions or conditions of use or warnings.".

SEC. 11. WITHDRAWAL OF THE REGULATIONS AND NOTICE.

The advance notice of proposed rulemaking concerning dietary supplements published in the Federal Register of June 18, 1993 (58 FR 33690-33700) is null and void and of no force or effect insofar as it applies to dietary supplements. The Secretary of Health and Human Services shall publish a notice in the Federal Register to revoke the item declared to be null and void and of no force or effect under subsection (a).

SEC. 12. COMMISSION ON DIETARY SUPPLEMENT LABELS.

(a) ESTABLISHMENT.—There shall be established as an independent agency within the executive branch a commission to be known as the Commission on Dietary Supplement Labels (hereafter in this section referred to as the "Commission").

(b) MEMBERSHIP.—

(1) COMPOSITION.—The Commission shall be composed of 7 members who shall be appointed by the President.

(2) EXPERTISE REQUIREMENT.—The members of the Commision shall consist of individuals with expertise and experience in dietary supplements and in the manufacture, regulation, distribution, and use of such supplements. At least three of the members of the Commission shall be qualified by scientific training and experience to evaluate the benefits to health of the use of dietary supplements and one of such three members shall have experience in pharmacognosy, medical botany, traditional herbal medicine, or other related sciences. Members and staff of the Commission shall be without bias on the issue of dietary supplements.

(c) FUNCTIONS OF THE COMMISSION.—The Commission shall conduct a study on, and provide recommendations for, the regulation of label claims and statements for dietary supplements, including the use of literature in connection with the sale of dietary supplements and procedures for the evaluation of such claims. In making such recommendations, the Commission shall evaluate how best to provide truthful, scientifically valid, and not misleading information to consumers so that such consumers may make informed and appropriate health care choices for themselves and their families.

(d) ADMINISTRATIVE POWERS OF THE COMMISSION—

(1) HEARINGS.—The Commission may hold hearings, sit and act at such times and places, take such testimony, and receive such evidence as the Commission considers advisable to carry out the purposes of this section.

(2) INFORMATION FROM FEDERAL AGENCIES.—The Commission may secure directly from any Federal department or agency such information as the Commission considers necessary to carry out the provisions of this section.

(3) AUTHORIZATION OF APPROPRIATIONS.—There are authorized to be appropriated such sums as may be necessary to carry out this section.

(e) REPORTS AND RECOMMENDATIONS.—

(1) FINAL REPORT REQUIRED.—Not later than 24 months after the date of enactment of this Act, the Commission shall prepare and submit to the President and to the Congress a final report on the study required by this section.

(2) RECOMMENDATIONS.—The report described in paragraph (1) shall contain such recommendations, including recommendations for legislation, as the Commission deems appropriate.

(3) ACTION ON RECOMMENDATIONS.—Within 90 days of the issuance of the report under paragraph (1), the Secretary of Health and Human Services shall publish in the Federal Register a notice of any recommendation of Commission for changes in regulations of the Secretary for the regulation of dietary supplements and shall include in such notice a notice of proposed rulemaking on such changes together with an opportunity to present views on such changes. Such rulemaking shall be completed not later than 2 years after the date of the issuance of such report. If such rulemaking is not completed on or before the expiration of such 2 years, regulations of the Secretary published in 59 FR 395-426 on January 4, 1994, shall not be in effect.

SEC. 13. OFFICE OF DIETARY SUPPLEMENTS.

(a) IN GENERAL.—Title IV of the Public Health Service Act is amended by inserting after section 485B (42 U.S.C. 287c-3) the following:

"Subpart 4—Office of Dietary Supplements

"SEC. 485C. DIETARY SUPPLEMENTS.

"(a) ESTABLISHMENT.—The Secretary shall establish an Office of Dietary Supplements within the National Institutes of Health.

"(b) PURPOSE.—The purposes of the Office are—

"(1) to explore more fully the potential role of dietary supplements as a significant part of the efforts of the United States to improve health care; and

"(2) to promote scientific study of the benefits of dietary supplements in maintaining health and preventing chronic disease and other health-related conditions.

"(c) DUTIES.—The Director of the Office of Dietary Supplements shall—

"(1) conduct and coordinate scientific research within the National Institutes of Health relating to dietary supplements and the extent to which the use of dietary supplements can limit or reduce the risk of diseases such as heart disease, cancer, birth defects, osteoporosis, cataracts, or prostatism;

"(2) collect and compile the results of scientific research relating to dietary supplements, including scientific data from foreign sources or the Office of Alternative Medicine;

"(3) serve as the principal advisor to the Secretary and to the Assistant Secretary for Health and provide advice to the Director of the National Institutes of Health, the Director of the Centers for Disease Control and Prevention, and the Commissioner of Food and Drugs on issues relating to dietary supplements including—

"(A) dietary intake regulations;

"(B) the safety of dietary supplements;

"(C) claims characterizing the relationship between—

"(i) dietary supplements; and

"(ii)(I) prevention of disease or other health-related conditions; and

"(II) maintenance of health; and

"(D) scientific issues arising in connection with the labeling and composition of dietary supplements;

"(4) compile a database of scientific research on dietary supplements and individual nutrients; and

"(5) coordinate funding relating to dietary supplements for the National Institutes of Health.

"(d) DEFINITION.—As used in this section, the term 'dietary supplement' has the meaning given the term in section 201(ff) of the Federal Food, Drug, and Cosmetic Act.

"(e) AUTHORIZATION OF APPROPRIATIONS.—There are authorized to be appropriated to carry out this section $5,000,000 for fiscal year 1994 and such sums as may be necessary for each subsequent fiscal year.".

(b) CONFORMING AMENDMENT.—Section 401(b)(2) of the Public Health Service Act (42 U.S.C. 281(b)(2)) is amended by adding at the end the following:

"(E) The Office of Dietary Supplements.".

Approved October 25, 1994.

Appendix B

Recommendations of the Canadian Standing Committee on Health

Definitions

Health Canada, in conjunction with a new separate NHP Expert Advisory Committee, set out an appropriate definition of NHPs and amend the Food and Drugs Act accordingly.

Health Canada, in conjunction with the new NHP Expert Advisory Committee, examine the status of bulk herbs for legislative purposes.

Expertise and Regulatory Structure

The Government give consideration to the advisability of creating a new regulatory authority for NHPs that reports directly to the Assistant Deputy Minister of the Health Protection Branch.

The structure for this new regulatory authority be established within the next six months and be permanently staffed by individuals with expertise and experience in the field of NHPs.

The selection of personnel be agreeable to both government and NHP stakeholders.

When necessary, working groups reflecting the various segments that make up the NHP category be set up to advise the new regulatory authority.

All relevant inspection personnel be provided with training specific to NHPs.

The necessary process to amend the Food and Drugs Act not delay in any way the implementation of the regulatory and administrative changes that can proceed at this time.

An Expert Advisory Committee be established immediately to assist Health Canada in the general and specific tasks necessary to design a new NHP regulatory environment.

Volpe, Joseph (Chair). November 1998. Natural health products: A new vision. Report on the Standing Committee on Health.

This Expert Advisory Committee review the reestablishment options for an NHP section with research and laboratory capacities and report its findings to Health Canada.

The selection of members for the Expert Advisory Committee be agreeable to both NHP stakeholders and Health Canada.

Safety

The new regulatory authority assume primary responsibility for assessing safety of products.

General safety protocols be developed by the Expert Advisory Committee based on EAC judgments of reasonable evidence.

When necessary, this regulatory authority establish appropriate working groups to assess the safety of specific products.

Quality/Good Manufacturing Practices

Health Canada, in collaboration with the NHP industry, establish appropriate GMP guidelines reflective of the different nature of NHPs.

GMP standards for NHPs include specific quality control and testing for herbal products.

Manufacturers, packagers, importers, and distributors of NHPs, whether located in Canada or abroad, be obliged to hold valid establishment licenses.

Inspection activities be performed consistently and on a regular basis by inspectors knowledgeable about the products.

Efficacy

NHPs be allowed to make health claims, including structure-function claims, risk-reduction claims, and treatment claims.

Claims be assessed to ensure that there is reasonable evidence supporting the claim.

The evidence not be limited to double-blind clinical trials but also include other types of evidence such as generally accepted and traditional references, professional consensus, other types of clinical trials, and other clinical or scientific evidence.

The evidence required vary depending on the type of claim being made, with different evidence being required for structure/function claims and risk-reduction claims for minor self-limiting conditions than for therapeutic or treatment claims.

The label indicates clearly the type of evidence used to support the claim.

Product Licensing

The new product licensing framework be based on a risk management approach that emphasizes the margin of safety associated with a particular product.

Health Canada, in conjunction with the Expert Advisory Committee, establish categories within the NHP class to determine what level of regulation is appropriate for a particular product.

A product licensing system based on monographs be used when they are available. Such a system should rely on a premarket approval process and the regulator should have a short period of time (for example, thirty days) to review the application.

Health Canada, in conjunction with the Expert Advisory Committee, establish procedures to create new Canadian monographs based on work already accomplished in other countries.

Manufacturers of products that do not have monographs be required to provide evidence to Health Canada before a product is marketed. The level of evidence would be consistent with the margin of safety associated with the product.

The level of postmarket monitoring be based on the margin of safety associated with the product and include an NHP adverse event reporting system for industry and an adverse reaction hotline for practitioners and the general public.

Certain lower safety products be made available to consumers with appropriate warnings and other lower safety products be made available only with practitioner intervention.

The new framework be phased in over a period of months to allow sufficient time for the stakeholders and the regulator to review the current DIN system and conform to the new regulations.

Labeling

Health Canada consult with its new separate NHP Expert Advisory Committee to determine what information is to be included on the labeling, consisting of, at a minimum, the items recommended by the Advisory Panel on Natural Health Products.

NHP labeling provide consumers with all relevant information needed to make informed choices.

NHP labeling be standardized to provide clear and consistent product information.

Section 3 and Schedule A of the Food and Drugs Act

Health Canada immediately initiate a review of the diseases listed in Schedule A to ensure that only appropriate diseases are included and, where relevant, specific diseases be exempted by regulation from the broad terms found in Schedule A.

Health Canada, subsequently, conduct a study with the participation of representatives from consumer groups, the food, natural health products and pharmaceutical industries, and health practitioners to determine whether subsections 3(1) and (2) of the Food and Drugs Act or all of the diseases listed in Schedule A should be deleted.

Importation of Human-Use Drugs for Personal Use

When the new regulatory framework is implemented, the personal importation policy be reviewed by Health Canada and the Expert Advisory Committee to determine if it is still appropriate and to outline permissible changes.

Cost Recovery

Health Canada conduct a review analyzing the impact of the overall cost recovery policy on the different segments of the NHP industry.

The NHP industry stakeholders be consulted in the establishment of the most appropriate fee structure and amount.

As a result of this review, the existing fee levels be reexamined if necessary.

Appeal Process

As part of the immediate process for NHPs, Health Canada work with stakeholders to establish appropriate, accessible and effective appeal processes for relevant policies and possible inclusion into a revised regulatory and legislative framework.

Informed Choice

Health Canada immediately utilize existing formats and forums for more open and transparent communication on NHPs with the broader public and practitioners.

Communication efforts include details about decisions and actions regarding NHP products (removal from market, change of status, etc.).

Relevant consumer, industry, and practitioner groups be consulted on a regular basis about the nature of the required information.

The federal government research bodies, including Health Canada, begin immediately to encourage research on NHPs. This could include studies focusing on the interactions of herbal products with conventional medications as well as studies that explore different uses by various groups in Canada.

Health Canada undertake, through its various established avenues, the dissemination of the resulting information to health care professionals and consumers.

NHP Practitioners

Health Canada inform its provincial and territorial counterparts of the regulatory changes with regard to NHPs and of the concerns raised by practitioners.

Enforcement

The new regulatory framework for NHPs be enforced in a regular and consistent manner and done in conjunction with education.

Sufficient resources be provided for enforcement activities.

Aboriginal Healers

If a product that is extemporaneously compounded for a particular person is not exempted from the regulatory framework, that such a product be exempted.

Plant Conservation

Health Canada work with Foreign Affairs and International Trade to ensure that existing International Agreements that currently protect biological diversity are not violated and that additional strategies are developed if needed to prevent depletion of these valuable health resources.

Transition

The interim enforcement policy regarding NHPs continue to be applied until the new framework is in place.

The Minister appoint, immediately, a transition team responsible for ensuring that the new framework is established quickly.

Appendix C

Abbreviations and Acronyms

AARP	American Association of Retired Persons
ACT UP	AIDS Coalition to Unleash Power
AESGP	Association of the European Self-Medication Industry
BATF	Bureau of Alcohol, Tobacco, and Firearms
BfArM	Federal Institute for Drugs and Medical Devices/*Bundesinstitut für Arzneimittel und Medizinprodukte* (Germany)
CFSAN	Center for Food Safety and Applied Nutrition
CGMP	Current Good Manufacturing Practices
DIN	Drug Identification Number (Canada)
DSHEA	Dietary Supplement Health and Education Act
EAC	Expert Advisory Committee (Canada)
EAPC	European-American Phytomedicines Coalition
EMEA	European Agency for the Evaluation of Medicinal Products
FDA	Food and Drug Administration
FDC Act	Food, Drug, and Cosmetic Act
FTC	Federal Trade Commmission
GAO	General Accounting Office
GMP	good manufacturing practices
GRAS	generally recognized as safe
GRASE	generally recognized as safe and effective
GSL	General Sale List (United Kingdom)
HACCP	Hazard Analysis and Critical Control Points
HHS	Health and Human Services
IBIDS	International Bibliographic Information on Dietary Supplements
JAMA	*Journal of the American Medical Association*
MAO	monoamine oxidase enzyme
MCA	Medicines Control Agency (United Kingdom)
MOU	memorandum of understanding
MRA	mutual recognition agreement
NCCAM	National Center for Complementary and Alternative Medicine
NDA	New Drug Application
NEJM	*New England Journal of Medicine*
NHP	natural health product (Canada)

NHPD	Natural Health Products Directorate (Canada)
NIH	National Institutes of Health
NLEA	Nutrition Labeling and Education Act
NNRTI	nonnucleoside reverse transcriptase inhibitors
NREA	Nutraceutical Research and Education Act
ODS	Office of Dietary Supplements
ONHP	Office of Natural Health Products (Canada)
OTC	over-the-counter drug
P	Pharmacy Medicine (United Kingdom)
PI	Protease Inhibitors
POM	Prescription Only Medicine (United Kingdom)
RDA	Recommended Daily Allowance
SSRI	selective serotonin reuptake inhibitor
TEA	time and extent application
THM	traditional herbal medicine (Canada)
TPP	Therapeutic Products Programme (Canada)
U.K.	United Kingdom
U.S.	United States of America
WHO	World Health Organization

Notes

Chapter 1

1. Eisenberg, David M., Roger B. Davis, Susan L. Ettner, Scott Appel, Sonja Wilkey, Maria Van Rompany, Ronald C. Kessler. 1998. Trends in alternative medicine use in the United States 1990-1997. *JAMA* 280(18):1569-1575.

2. Linde, Klaus, Gilbert Ramirez, Cynthia D. Mulrow, Andrej Pauls, Wolfgang Weidenhammer, and Dieter Melchart. 1996. St. John's wort for depression—An overview and meta-analysis of randomised clinical trials. *British Medical Journal* 313(7052):253-258.

3. Hypericum Depression Trial Study Group. 2002. Effect of *Hypericum perforatum* (St. John's wort) in major depressive disorder: A randomized controlled trial. *Journal of the American Medical Association* 287(14), p. 1813.

4. Food and Drug Administration. 1997. Dietary supplements containing ephedrine alkaloids; proposed rule. *Federal Register* 62(107):30677-30724.

5. General Accounting Office. 1999. Dietary supplements: Uncertainties in analyses underlying FDA's proposed rule on ephedrine alkaloids. Report to the Chairman and Ranking Minority Member, Committee on Science, House of Representatives. GAO/HEHS/GGD-99-90.

Chapter 2

1. Schwartz, John. FDA targets untrue product claims; report lists 500 unsubstantiated statements on vitamins, dietary supplements. *The Washington Post,* July 30, 1993, p. A19.

2. Food and Drug Act of 1906, ch. 3915, 34 Stat. 768 (repealed 1938).

3. Fink, Joseph L. and Simonsmeier, Larry M. 1985. Laws governing pharmacy. In: *Remington's Pharmaceutical Sciences,* Alfonso R. Gennaro ed., Seventeenth edition, pp. 1890-1916. Easton, PA: Mack.

4. Ibid.

5. Cavers, David F. 1939. *The Food, Drug, and Cosmetic Act of 1938: Its Legislative History and Its Substantive Provisions.*

6. Public Law 75-717, 52 Stat. 1040 (1938) (codified as amended at 21 U.S.C. Sections 301-395 [1994]).

7. Cataxinos, Edgar R. 1995. Regulation of herbal medications in the United States: Germany provides a model for reform. *Utah Law Review* Rev. 561.

8. Hutt, Peter B. and Merrill, Richard A. 1991. *Food and Drug Law: Cases and Materials,* Second Edition. Westbury, NY: Foundation Press.

9. Public Law 87-781, 76 Stat. 780 (codified as amended at 21 U.S.C. Sections 301-395 [1994]).

10. Cataxinos, Edgar R. 1995. Regulation of herbal medications in the United States: Germany provides a model for reform. *Utah Law Review* Rev. 561, p. 564.

11. Manual of Patent Examining Procedure, section 706.03(a): "a thing occurring in nature, which is substantially unaltered, is not a 'manufacture' " and is therefore not patentable matter.

12. Food and Drug Administration. 1972. *Federal Register* 37:9464.

13. Tyler, Varro E. 1986. Plant drugs in the twenty-first century. *Economic Botany* 40:279-281.

14. Personal communication. Bob Eshelman, Food and Drug Administration, Center for Drug Evaluation and Research, Office of Compliance, Division of Labeling and Non-Prescription Drug Compliance, OTC Compliance Team. April 27, 2000.

15. Cataxinos, Edgar R. 1995. Regulation of herbal medications in the United States: Germany provides a model for reform. *Utah Law Review* Rev. 561.

16. H401-13. FDA's continuing failure to regulate health claims for foods. October 31, November 9, 1989.

17. Nutrition labeling. *Congressional Quarterly Almanac 1989.* pp. 179-180.

18. Standardized Food Labeling Ordered. *Congressional Quarterly Almanac 1990,* pp. 575-576.

19. Public Law 101-535, 104 Stat. 2353 (codified as amended at 21 U.S.C. Sections 301, 321, 337, 343, 345, 371 [1994]).

20. Cataxinos, Edgar R. 1995. Regulation of herbal medications in the United States: Germany provides a model for reform. *Utah Law Review* Rev. 561.

21. Standardized food labeling ordered. *Congressional Quarterly Almanac 1990,* pp. 575-576 (quote is on p. 576).

22. Drug makers to pay fees for FDA reviews. *Congressional Quarterly Almanac 1992,* pp. 418-421 (quote is on p. 421).

23. Israelsen, L., President, Utah Natural Products Alliance. Oral testimony presented to the Commission on Dietary Supplement Labels. March 8, 1996. Salt Lake City, UT.

24. Hatch cites his experience, but his campaign needs contributions fast if it is to keep going. *The Wall Street Journal,* January 19, 2000, p. A24.

25. Murray, Frank. Senator Orrin G. Hatch is our man of the year. *Better Nutrition for Today's Living,* October 1993, pp. 6-7.

26. Wittes, Benjamin. FDA exemption sought for self-help medicines. *Legal Times,* October 7, 1994.

27. Blonz, Edward. Pending FDA regulation on supplements sparks protests. *The San Diego Union-Tribune,* August 12, 1993, p. 1, Food section.

28. Dietary supplement bill faces a tough time in the house. *Congressional Quarterly,* August 20, 1994, p. 2461.

29. Blonz, Edward. Pending FDA regulation on supplements sparks protests. *The San Diego Union-Tribune,* August 12, 1993, p. 1, Food section.

30. Wittes, Benjamin. FDA exemption sought for self-help medicines. *Legal Times,* October 7, 1994, p. 2.

31. Blonz, Edward. Pending FDA regulation on supplements sparks protests. *The San Diego Union-Tribune,* August 12, 1993, p. 1, Food section.

32. Wittes, Benjamin. FDA exemption sought for self-help medicines. *Legal Times,* October 7, 1994, p. 2.

33. Ibid.

34. Ibid.

35. Jacobson, Michael F. Perspective on dietary supplements. *Los Angeles Times,* November 22, 1993, p. 7, Home section.

36. Henry A. Waxman in Regulation of dietary supplements: Hearing before the Subcommittee on Health and Environment, Committee on Energy and Commerce, House of Representatives, July 29, 1993.

37. Kingdon, John. 1984. *Agendas, Alternatives and Public Policies.* Boston: Little, Brown.

38. Goodsell, Charles. 1994. *The Case for Bureaucracy,* Third Edition.

39. David A. Kessler in Regulation of dietary supplements: Hearing before the Subcommittee on Health and Environment, Committee on Energy and Commerce, House of Representatives, July 29, 1993, p. 63.

40. Kingdon, John. 1984. *Agendas, Alternatives and Public Policies.* Boston: Little, Brown.

41. Senate panel votes to restrict diet supplement regulations 1994. *Congressional Quarterly* 52(19):1228.

42. Drug makers to pay fees for FDA reviews. *Congressional Quarterly Almanac 1992,* pp. 418-421.

43. Silverglade, Bruce A. Without regulation, charlatans prosper; concern over proposed legislation to undermine regulations for scientific claims proffered by dietary supplement industry. *Insight on the News,* September 5, 1994.

44. Hatch, Orrin G., Robert N. Mayer, and Debra L. Scammon. 1994. Congress versus the Food and Drug Administration: How one government health agency harms the public health. *Journal of Public Policy and Marketing* 13(1):151-152.

45. Wittes, Benjamin. FDA exemption sought for self-help medicines. *Legal Times,* October 7, 1994, p. 2.

46. Orrin G. Hatch in Regulation of dietary supplements: Hearing before the Subcommittee on Health and Environment, Committee on Energy and Commerce, House of Representatives, July 29, 1993.

47. 21 U.S.C. Section 343(r)(3)(B)(i) (1994).

48. Orrin G. Hatch in Regulation of dietary supplements: Hearing before the Subcommittee on Health and Environment, Committee on Energy and Commerce, House of Representatives, July 29, 1993, p. 4.

49. Ibid.

50. Bruce Silverglade quoting the Nutrition Health Alliance in Hearing of the Subcommittee on Health and Environment, Committee on Energy and Commerce, House of Representatives, July 29, 1993, p. 276.

51. Supplement rules pending; panel delays action. *Congressional Quarterly,* November 20, 1993, p. 3204.

52. The Tan Sheet. *The News This Week,* May 3, 1993, pp. 8-10.

53. David A. Kessler in Hearing of the Subcommittee on Health and Environment, Committee on Energy and Commerce, House of Representatives, July 29, 1993.

54. Supplement rules pending; panel delays action. *Congressional Quarterly,* November 20, 1993, p. 3204.

55. Orrin G. Hatch in Regulation of dietary supplements: Hearing before the Subcommittee on Health and Environment, Committee on Energy and Commerce, House of Representatives, July 29, 1993, p. 7.

56. David A. Kessler in Regulation of dietary supplements: Hearing before the Subcommittee on Health and Environment, Committee on Energy and Commerce, House of Representatives, July 29, 1993, p. 64.

57. Ibid, p. 69.

58. Schwartz, John. FDA targets untrue product claims; report lists 500 unsubstantiated statements on vitamins, dietary supplements. *The Washington Post,* July 30, 1993, p. A19.

59. David A. Kessler in Regulation of dietary supplements: Hearing before the Subcommittee on Health and Environment, Committee on Energy and Commerce, House of Representatives, July 29, 1993.

60. Schwartz, John. FDA targets untrue product claims; report lists 500 unsubstantiated statements on vitamins, dietary supplements. *The Washington Post,* July 30, 1993, p. A19.

61. David A. Kessler in Regulation of dietary supplements: Hearing before the Subcommittee on Health and Environment, Committee on Energy and Commerce, House of Representatives, July 29, 1993.

62. Schwartz, John. FDA targets untrue product claims; report lists 500 unsubstantiated statements on vitamins, dietary supplements. *The Washington Post,* July 30, 1993, p. A19.

63. Hatch, Orrin G., Robert N. Mayer, and Debra L. Scammon. 1994. Congress versus the Food and Drug Administration: How one government health agency harms the public health. *Journal of Public Policy and Marketing* 13(1):151-152.

64. Blonz, Edward. Pending FDA regulation on supplement sparks protest. *The San Diego Union-Tribune,* August 12, 1993, p. 1, Food section.

65. Senate panel votes to restrict diet supplement regulations. 1994. *Congressional Quarterly* 52(19):1228.

66. Deal struck on regulation of dietary supplements. 1994. *Congressional Quarterly* 52(39):2888.

67. Supplement rules pending; panel delays action. *Congressional Quarterly,* November 20, 1993, p. 3204.

68. Senate tries to delay diet supplement rules. *Congressional Quarterly Almanac 1993,* pp. 371-372.

69. Ibid.

70. Jacobson, Michael F. Perspective on dietary supplements. *Los Angeles Times,* November 22, 1993, p. 7, Home section.

71. Ibid.

72. Ibid.

73. Senate panel votes to restrict diet supplement regulations. 1994. *Congressional Quarterly* 52(19):1228.

74. Ibid.

75. Ibid.

76. Ibid.

77. Ibid.

78. Dietary Supplement Health and Education Act. 1994. Public Law 103-417, Section 485C(b)(2).

79. Senate panel votes to restrict diet supplement regulations. 1994. *Congressional Quarterly* 52(19):1228.

80. Deal struck on regulation of dietary supplements. 1994. *Congressional Quarterly* 52(39):2888.

81. Ibid.

82. Ibid.

83. Bill Kolasky, outside counsel for the Council for Responsible Nutrition, quoted in Supplement industry launches final push for legislation. *Food Chemical News,* September 26, 1994, p. 29.

84. Deal struck on regulation of dietary supplements. 1994. *Congressional Quarterly* 52(39):2888.

85. Council for Responsible Nutrition. <http://www.crnusa.org/shellgovt000001. html>.

86. Wittes, Benjamin. FDA exemption sought for self-help medicines. *Legal Times,* October 7, 1994, p. 2.

87. Silverglade, Bruce A. Without regulation, charlatans prosper; concern over proposed legislation to undermine regulations for scientific claims proffered by dietary supplement industry. *Insight on the News.* September 5, 1994, pp. 20-22.

88. Clare Hasler quoted in Sweetener group testing supplement act waters. *Food Chemical News.* November 21, 1994, p. 50.

89. Dietary Supplement Health and Education Act. 1994. Public Law 103-417.

90. Food and Drug Administration. 1998. Cholestin from Beijing WBL Peking University Biotech Co. Ltd., Beijing, China. Import Bulletin #61-B02, revised March 27, 1998.

91. U.S. District Court for District of Utah, Central Division. 1998. Order. Case No. 2:97CV 0262 K. *Pharmanex Inc. v. Shalala and Friedman.*

92. *Pharmanex Inc. v. Shalala,* 35 F. Supp. 2d 1341 (Cent. Dist. Utah 1999).

93. Ibid.

94. Ibid, Discussion, Section 2, p. 7.

95. FDA appealing Utah federal court ruling on Cholestin. 1999. *Food Chemical News* 41(11):27.

96. Food and Drug Administration. Letter to The Honorable Dan Burton, Chairman, House Committee on Government Reform. February 1, 2002.

97. Commission on Dietary Supplement Labels. 1997. *Report on the Commission on Dietary Supplement Labels.*

98. Office of the Federal Register. 1997. Code of Federal Regulations. Procedures for classifying OTC drugs as generally recognized as safe and effective and

not misbranded, and for establishing monographs. Title 21: Food and drugs, part 330.10 rev. Washington, DC: U.S. Government Printing Office.

99. Office of the Federal Register. 1997. Code of Federal Regulations. Adequate and well-controlled studies. Title 21: Food and drugs, part 314.126 rev. Washington, DC: U.S. Government Printing Office.

100. Manual of Patent Examining Procedure Section 706.03(a): "a thing occurring in nature, which is substantially unaltered, is not a 'manufacture' " and is therefore not patentable matter.

101. Section 201(p) 21 U.S.C. 321 (p).

102. Food and Drug Administration. 1999. Additional criteria and procedures for classifying over-the-counter drugs as generally recognized as safe and effective and not misbranded. *Federal Register* 64(243):71062-71082.

103. Food and Drug Administration. 2002. Additional criteria and procedures for classifying over-the-counter drugs as generally safe and effective and not misbranded. *Federal Register* 67(15):3060-3076. 21 CFR Section 330.14.

104. Commission on Dietary Supplement Labels. 1997. *Report on the Commission on Dietary Supplement Labels,* p. 52.

105. Ibid, p. 57.

106. Ibid.

107. Ibid.

108. Ibid, p. xi.

109. Food and Drug Administration. 2000. Draft guidance for industry: Botanical drug products.

110. Ibid, p. 1.

111. Federal Trade Commission Act, 5 U.S.C. 45.

112. Federal Trade Commission. 1994. Enforcement policy statement on food advertising. *Federal Register* 59:28388-28396.

113. Federal Trade Commission. 1983. Advertising substantiation program; request for comment. Policy statement regarding advertising substantiation. *Federal Register* 48:10471-10475.

114. Food and Drug Administration. 1999. Agency information collection activities: proposed collection; comment request; premarket notification for a new dietary ingredient. *Federal Register* 64(26):6364-6365.

115. Food and Drug Administration. 1999. Agency information collection activities; submission for OMB review; comment request and correction; premarket notification for a new dietary ingredient. *Federal Register* 64(88):24660-24661.

116. 42 U.S.C. 264.

117. Public Law 104-134, amended by Public Law 104-180.

118. Food and Drug Administration. 1998. Draft guidance for industry; exports and imports under the FDA Export Reform and Enhancement Act of 1996. *Federal Register* 63:32219-32235.

119. Office of the Federal Register. 1997. *Code of Federal Regulations.* Current good manufacturing practice in manufacturing, packing or holding human food. Title 21: Food and drugs, part 110 rev. Washington, DC: U.S. Government Printing Office.

120. Food and Drug Administration. 1997. Current Good Manufacturing Practice in Manufacturing, Packing, or Holding Dietary Supplements; Proposed Rule. *Federal Register* 62(25):5699-5709 (quote on p. 5701).

121. Food and Drug Administration. 1998. Good Manufacturing Practices for Dietary Supplements Working Group of the Food Advisory Committee; notice of meeting. *Federal Register* 68(188):51942.

122. Food and Drug Administration. 1999. Dietary supplements; Center for Food Safety and Applied Nutrition; public meeting. *Federal Register* 64(117):32830-32831 (quote on p. 32830).

123. Ibid.

124. Ibid.

125. Food and Drug Administration. Letter to The Honorable Dan Burton, Chairman, House Committee on Government Reform. February 1, 2002.

126. Dietary Supplement Health and Education Act. 1994. Public Law 103-417, Section 12(c).

127. Commission on Dietary Supplement Labels. 1997. *Report on the Commission on Dietary Supplement Labels.*

128. McCaleb, Rob and Mark Blumenthal. 1997. President's Commission on Dietary Supplement Labels issues final report. *HerbalGram* 41:24-26.

129. Dietary Supplement Health and Education Act. 1994. Public Law 103-417, Section 6.

130. Ibid.

131. Food and Drug Administration. 1998. Regulations on statements made for dietary supplements concerning the effect of the product on the structure or function of the body. *Federal Register* 63(82):23624-23632.

132. Ibid, pp. 23626-23627.

133. Food and Drug Administration. 2000. Regulations on statements made for dietary supplements concerning the effect of the product on the structure or function of the body. *Federal Register* 65(4):1000-1050. Codified 21 CFR 101.93(g).

134. Food and Drug Administration. 1999. Regulations on statements made for dietary supplements concerning the effect of the product on the structure or function of the body; public meeting. *Federal Register* 64(130):36824-36826.

135. Ibid, p. 36824.

136. 21 CFR 101.14(a)(6).

137. Food and Drug Administration. 1998. Regulations on statements made for dietary supplements concerning the effect of the product on the structure or function of the body. *Federal Register* 63(82):23624-23632 (quote on pp. 23625-23626).

138. Food and Drug Administration. 1999. Regulations on statements made for dietary supplements concerning the effect of the product on the structure or function of the body; public meeting. *Federal Register* 64(130):36824-36826 (quote on p. 36825).

139. Food and Drug Administration. 1998. Regulations on statements made for dietary supplements concerning the effect of the product on the structure or function of the body. *Federal Register* 63(82):23624-23632 (quote on p. 23626).

140. Food and Drug Administration. 2000. Regulations on statements made for dietary supplements concerning the effect of the product on the structure or function of the body. *Federal Register* 65(4):1000-1050.

141. Food and Drug Administration. 1998. Regulations on statements made for dietary supplements concerning the effect of the product on the structure or function of the body. *Federal Register* 63(82):23624-23632 (quote on p. 23627).

142. Food and Drug Administration. 2000. Regulations on statements made for dietary supplements concerning the effect of the product on the structure or function of the body. *Federal Register* 65(4):1000-1050 (quote on p. 1000).

143. F.D.A. draws fire for a rule on supplements and pregnancy. *The New York Times*. February 4, 2000, A16.

144. Food and Drug Administration. FDA statement concerning structure/function rule and pregnancy claims. HHS Statement, February 9, 2000. <http://vm.cfsan.fda.gov/~lrd/hhssupp3.html>.

145. Food and Drug Administration. 2000. Regulations on statements made for dietary suplements concerning the effect of the product on the structure or function of the body. *Federal Register* 65(4):1000-1050 (quote on p. 1001).

146. Food and Drug Administration. 1999. Agency information collection activities: proposed collection; comment request; food labeling; notification procedures for statements on dietary supplements. *Federal Register* 64(23):5664-5665.

147. Food and Drug Administration. 1999. Agency information collection activities; submission for OMB review; comment request; food labeling; notification procedures for statements on dietary supplements. *Federal Register* 64(88):24659-24660.

148. Commission on Dietary Supplement Labels. 1997. *Report on the Commission on Dietary Supplement Labels,* pp. ix-x.

149. Food and Drug Administration. 1998. Dietary supplements; comments on Report of the Commission on Dietary Supplement Labels. *Federal Register* 63(82):23633-23637.

150. Nutrition Labeling and Education Act. 1990. Public Law 101-535.

151. Food and Drug Administration Modernization Act of 1997. Public Law 105-115.

152. *Pearson v. Shalala,* 164 F.3d 650 (D.C. Cir. 1999).

153. Food and Drug Administration. 1999. Food labeling: Health claims and label statements for dietary supplements; strategy for implementation of Pearson court decision. *Federal Register* 64(230):67289-67291.

154. Food and Drug Administration. 2000. Food labeling; health claims and label statements for dietary supplements; update to strategy for implementation of Pearson court decision. *Federal Register* 65(195):59855-59857.

155. Food and Drug Administration. 1999. Guidance for industry: Significant scientific agreement in the review of health claims for conventional foods and dietary supplements.

156. Food and Drug Administration. 2000. Food labeling; health claims and label statements for dietary supplements; update to strategy for implementation of Pearson court decision. *Federal Register* 65(195):59855-59857.

157. Food and Drug Administration. 2001. Letter regarding a health claim for folic acid and neural tube defects.

158. http://www.emord.com/lawsuits.htm.

159. Foster, S. (Ed.) 1992. *Herbs of Commerce.* Bethesda, MD: American Herbal Products Association.

160. Food and Drug Administration. 1998. Food labeling: Statement of identity, nutrition labeling and ingredient labeling of dietary supplements; compliance policy guide, revocation. *Federal Register* 63(108):30615-30621.

161. Federal Trade Commission Act, 5 U.S.C. 45.

162. Federal Trade Commission. 1994. Enforcement policy statement on food advertising. *Federal Register* 59:28388-28396.

163. Federal Trade Commission. 1983. Advertising substantiation program; request for comment. Policy statement regarding advertising substantiation. *Federal Register* 48:10471-10475.

164. Commission on Dietary Supplement Labels. 1997. *Report on the Commission on Dietary Supplement Labels,* p. 47.

165. Ibid, p. 26.

166. Ibid, p. 21.

167. Office of Inspector General. 2001. Adverse event reporting for dietary supplements: An inadequate safety valve.

168. Ibid, p. iv.

169. Ibid, pp. ii-iii.

170. Food and Drug Administration. Dietary supplements; Center for Food Safety and Applied Nutrition strategy; public meeting. *Federal Register* 64(92):25889-25890 (quote on p. 25890).

171. Ibid.

172. Ibid.

173. Food and Drug Administration. January 2000. Dietary Supplement Strategy (Ten Year Plan).

174. Ibid, p. 1.

175. Ibid, p. 5.

176. HR 3001, 106th Congress, 1st Session, p. 1.

177. 21 U.S.C. 360ee(b)(3).

178. HR 3001, 106th Congress, 1st Session, p. 7, lines 12-16.

Chapter 3

1. European Association of Proprietary Medicine Manufacturers (AESGP). 1998. *Herbal medicinal products in the European Union.* European Commission.

2. Volpe, Joseph (Chair). November 1998. *Natural health products: A new vision.* Report of the Standing Committee on Health.

3. Ibid.

4. Ibid.

5. Health Canada. 1999. Transition team progress report I: A fresh vision for wellness, regulatory approach.

6. Health Canada. 2000. A fresh start: Final report of the ONHP transition team.

7. Health Canada. 2001. Health Minister Allan Rock announces measures to ensure Canadians make safe choices in natural health products.

8. CTV/Angus Reid Group Poll, August 1997.

9. *Canada Health Monitor.* June-July 1997. Survey 16. Forty-seven percent reported taking vitamins in the previous six months, 22 percent mineral supplements, 8 percent homeopathic products, 5 percent nutraceuticals, and 4 percent another product.

10. Health Canada. 2002. Regulatory impact analysis statement. Benefits and costs.

11. Health Protection Branch, Canada. 1990. *Traditional Herbal Medicines, Drugs Directorate Guideline.*

12. Bureau of Nonprescription Drugs, The Drugs Directorate, Canada. October 1995. *Policy Issues: Medicinal Herbs in Traditional Herbal Medicines.*

13. Health Protection Branch, Canada. 1990. *Homeopathic Preparations: Application for Drug Identification Numbers,* Drugs Directorate Guideline.

14. Health Canada. Natural health product regulations. *Canada Gazette,* December 22, 2001.

15. Schedule 705, proposed amendments to the Food and Drug Regulations.

16. Health Protection Branch, Canada. 1990. *Traditional Herbal Medicines, Drugs Directorate Guideline.*

17. Ibid.

18. Health Canada. A fresh start: Final report of the ONHP transition team. March 31, 2000. Page 30, Section 3.2.5(a).

19. Ibid, p. 30, Section 3.2.5(c).

20. Health Canada. Natural health product regulations. *Canada Gazette,* December 22, 2001. Page 5, Application (2).

21. Ibid, p. 5, Application (3).

22. Health Canada. A fresh start: Final report of the ONHP transition team. March 31, 2000. Page 32, Section 3.2.5(e).

23. Ibid, p. 30, Section 3.2.5(b).

24. Health Canada. Natural health product regulations. *Canada Gazette,* December 22, 2001. Pages 31-47, Part 4.

25. Food and Drugs Act and Regulations, Division 2, Part C.

26. Good Manufacturing Practices, Supplementary Guidelines for the Manufacture of Herbal Medicinal Products, Final Version, Drugs Directorate, Canada, 1996 (updated in 1998).

27. WHO Guidelines on the Assessment of Herbal Medicines.

28. Health Canada. 2002. Regulatory impact analysis statement. Site licensing (part 2 of the regulations).

29. Health Canada. 2002. Draft guidance on good manufacturing practices for natural health products.

30. Health Canada. 2002. Regulations impact analysis statement. Labelling and packaging (part 5 of the regulations).

31. Health Canada. Natural health product regulations. *Canada Gazette,* December 22, 2001. Pages 48-50, Part 5.

32. Health Canada. 2000. A fresh start: Final report of the ONHP transition team. Page 7.

33. Health Canada. Natural health product regulations. *Canada Gazette,* December 22, 2001. Pages 1 and 4, Interpretation (1).

34. Health Canada. 2002. Regulations Impact Analysis Statement. Adverse reactions (part 1 of the regulations).

Chapter 4

1. The Association of the European Self-Medication Industry (AESGP). 1998. *Herbal medicinal products in the European Union.* European Commission.

2. Law on Foodstuffs and Consumer Goods ("Lebensmittel-und Bedarfsgegenständegesetz" or "LMBG"), Section 1.

3. European Note for Guidance on Quality of Herbal Remedies; European Pharmacopoeia; and German Medicines Law, Section 26 (Arzneimittel-Prüfrichtlinien), May 5, 1995 implementing European Directive 91/507/EEC. (Bekanntmachung der Neufassung der Allgemeinen Verwaltungsvorschrift zur Anwendung der Arzneimittel Prüfrichtlinien vom 5. Mai 1995. *Bundesanzeiger* 1995;47 No. 96a, May 20, 1995.)

4. Keller, K. 1992. Results of the revision of herbal drugs in the Federal Republic of Germany with a special focus on risk aspects. *Zeitschrift fur Phytotherapie* 116:118.

5. Medicines Law of 1976, Section 25, Paragraph 7.

6. Bergner, Paul. 1994. German evaluation of herbal medicines. *Herbalgram,* 30:17,64

7. Ibid.

8. European Association of Proprietary Medicine Manufacturers (AESGP). 1998. *Herbal medicinal products in the European Union.* European Commission.

9. Medicines Law, Section 105, Paragraph 5c.

10. Medicines Law, Section 109a.

11. Allgemeine Verwaltungsvorschriften zur Anwendung der Arzneimittel Prüfrichtlinien vom 14. Dezember 1989. *Bundesanzeiger 1989;* 41 No. 243a of December 29, 1989.

12. Bekanntmachung der Neufassung der Allgemeinen Verwaltungsvorschrift zur Anwendung der Arzneimittel Prüfrichtlinien vom 5. Mai 1995. *Bundesanzeiger 1995;* 47 No. 96a, May 20, 1995.

13. Guidelines for Medicines Testing, Section 5. (Bekanntmachung der Neufassung der Allgemeinen Verwaltungsvorschrift zur Anwendung der Arzneimittel Prüfrichtlinien vom 5. Mai 1995. *Bundesanzeiger 1995;* 47 No. 96a, May 20, 1995.)

14. Medicines Law, Section 22, Paragraph 3a.

15. Pharmabetriebsverordnung (PharmBetrVO).

16. Fifth Amendment to the Medicines Law, *Federal Gazette,* August 16, 1994.

17. Law on Foodstuffs and Consumer Goods, Section 18, Article 1, Point 1.

18. European Association of Proprietary Medicine Manufacturers (AESGP). 1998. *Herbal medicinal products in the European Union.* European Commission.

19. Law on Foodstuffs and Consumer Goods, Section 17, Paragraph 1, Point 5a.

20. Law on Foodstuffs and Consumer Goods, Section 17, Paragraph 1, Point 5c.

21. European Directive 65/65/EEC, Article 2.4, Section 21, Paragraph 1 and Section 4, Paragraph 1.

22. European Directive 65/65/EEC, Article 2.5, Section 21, Paragraph 2, Point 1.

Chapter 5

1. The Association of the European Self-Medication Industry (AESGP). 1998. *Herbal medicinal products in the European Union.* European Commission.

2. Code de la Santé Publique, Article L.511.

3. Médicaments à base de plantes (September 1997). *Les Cahiers de l'Agence* no. 3. Agence du Médicament (this document replaced the previous Notice to Applicants published in the Bulletin officiel no. 90/22 bis.1990).

4. Code de la Santé Publique, Article L.512-5.

5. *Monograph plantes médicinales,* March 1991.

6. Décret 79-480 du 15 juin 1979 (J.O. du 22 juin 1979). Vente des plantes servant à la composition de boissons hygiéniques Loi du 21 juin 1941 (J.O. du 24 juin 1941). Vente au public de plantes médicinales inscrites à la Pharmacopée.

7. Circulaire 346 du 2 juillet 1979 (B.O.M.S. du 12 septembre 1979, 79/32) du Ministre de la Santé et de la Famille.

8. Code de la Santé Publique, Article L.601.

9. Code de la Santé Publique, Articles R.5128-5136.

10. Code de la Santé Publique, Article R.5133.

11. Médicaments à base de plantes (September 1997). *Les Cahiers de l'Agence* no. 3. Agence du Médicament (this document replaces the previous Notice to Applicants published in the Bulletin officiel no. 90/22 bis.1990).

12. Directive 92/27/EEC as implemented by Decree No. 94-19 of January 5, 1994 (published on January 9, 1994).

13. Directive 92/28/EEC as implemented by Decree No. 94-43 of January 18, 1994 (published on January 19, 1994) and by Decree No. 96-531 of June 14, 1996 (*Journal Official de la République Française,* June 16, 1996), modifying Articles R.5045 to 5055-4 of the Code de la Santé Publique.

14. Code de la Santé Publique, Article L.512-5.

15. Decree no. 95-284, March 14, 1995.

16. Mélanges de plantes autorisés à être vendus par les herboristes. Arrêté du 7 avril 1943 (J.O. du 4 mai 1943) modifié par Arrêté du 27 janvier 1959 (J.O. du 15 février 1959).

Chapter 6

1. The Association of the European Self-Medication Industry (AESGP). 1998. *Herbal medicinal products in the European Union.* European Commission.

2. UK Statutory Instrument 1994 No. 3144, The Medicines for Human Use (Marketing Authorisations, etc.) Regulations 1994.

3. Medicines Law 1968. London: HMSO, 1968.

4. Medicines Law 1968, Section 12(1).

5. Medicines Law 1968, Section 12(2).

6. Medicines Control Agency. A guide to what is a medicinal product. Medicines Law Leaflet MAL 8. London. December 1995.

7. Medicines Law 1968, Part II.

8. The Medicines Labelling (Amendment) Regulations 1992 (SI 1992/3273).

9. The Medicines Leaflets (Amendment) Regulations 1992 (SI 1992/3274).

10. The Medicines (Advertising) Regulations 1994 (SI 1994/1932).

11. The Medicines (Monitoring of Advertising) Regulation 1994 (SI 1994/1993).

12. The Medicines (Advertising) Amendment Regulations 1996 (SI 1996/1552).

13. The Medicines (Exemptions from Licences) (Special and Transitional Cases) Order 1971 (k).

14. The Medicines (Retail Sale or Supply of Herbal Remedies) Order 1977. London: HMSO, 1977 (Statutory Instrument: SI 1977 No. 2130).

Chapter 7

1. European Association of Proprietary Medicine Manufacturers (AESGP). 1998. *Herbal medicinal products in the European Union.* European Commission.

Chapter 8

1. Baldwin, Elaine and Anita Greene. 1997. St. John's wort study launched. National Institutes of Health.

2. Sclar, D.A., T.L. Skaer, L.M. Robison, and J.K. Stowers. 1998. Economic appraisal of antidepressant pharmacotherapy: Critical review of the literature and future directions. *Depression and Anxiety* 8 Suppl. 1:121-7.

3. Garattini, S., C. Barbui, and B. Saraceno. 1998. Antidepressant agents: From tricyclics to serotonin uptake inhibitors. *Psychological Medicine* 28(5):1169-1178 (quote on p. 1175).

4. Andrews, Edmund L. In Germany, humble herb is a rival to Prozac. *The New York Times.* September 9, 1997, C1.

5. Brody, Jane E. Personal Health column. *The New York Times.* September 10, 1997, C10.

6. Bratman, Steven. 1997. *Beat Depression with St. John's wort.* Rocklin, CA: Prima Publishing.

7. Carper, Jean. 1997. The Prozac of plants (St. John's wort—*Hypericum*). In: *Miracle Cures: Dramatic new scientific discoveries revealing the healing powers of herbs, vitamins, and other natural remedies.* New York: HarperCollins Publishers.

8. Brevoort, Peggy. 1998. The booming U.S. botanical market: A new overview. *Herbalgram* 44:33-46.

9. *Nutrition Business Journal.* 1999. *Third Annual Review of the Nutrition Industry* and *Data Book on the Nutrition Industry.*

10. Collado Campos, Manuel. Presented at the American Herbal Products Association's International Symposium on St. John's wort, Anaheim, California, March 16-17, 1998.

11. Overall supplement sales slightly up. *Natural Products Industry Insider,* March 11, 2002, p. 1.

12. Harrer, G., U. Schmidt, U. Kuhn, and A. Biller. 1999. Comparison of equivalence between the St. John's wort extract LoHyp-57 and fluoxetine. *Arzneimittel-Forschung.* 49(4):289-96.

13. Hansgen, K.D., and J. Vesper. 1996. Antidepressive Wirksamkeit eines hochdosierten *Hypericum*-Extraktes. *Muenchener Medizinische Wochenschrift* 138:35-39.

14. Witte, B., G. Harrer, T. Kaptan, H. Podzuweit, and U. Schmidt. 1995. Treatment of depressive symptoms with a high concentration *Hypericum* preparation. A multicenter placebo-controlled double-blind study. *Fortschritte der Medizin.* 113(28):404-408.

15. Hansgen, K.D., J. Vesper, and M. Ploch. 1994. Multicenter double-blind study examining the antidepressant effectiveness of the *Hypericum* extract LI 160. *Journal of Geriatric Psychiatry and Neurology* 7(Suppl. 1):S15-S18.

16. Harrer, G., and V. Schulz. 1994. Clinical investigation of the antidepressant effectiveness of *Hypericum. Journal of Geriatric Psychiatry and Neurology.* 7(Suppl. 1):S6-S8.

17. Harrer, G., W.D. Hübner, and H. Podzuweit. 1994. Effectiveness and tolerance of the *Hypericum* extract LI 160 in comparison with maprotiline: A multicenter double-blind study. *Journal of Geriatric Psychiatry and Neurology* 7(Suppl. 1):S24-S28.

18. Sommer, H., and G. Harrer. 1994. Placebo-controlled double-blind study examining the effectiveness of an *Hypericum* preparation in 105 mildly depressed patients. *Journal of Geriatric Psychiatry and Neurology.* 7(Suppl. 1):S9-S11.

19. Reh, C., P. Laux, and N. Schenk. 192. *Hypericum*—Extrakt bel Depressionen— eine wirksame Alternative. *Therapiewoche* 42:1576-1581.

20. Siegers, C.P., S. Biel, and K.P. Wilhelm. 1993. Phototoxicity caused by *Hypericum. Nervenheilkunde* 12:320-322.

21. De Smet, P.A., and W.A. Nolen. 1996. St. John's wort as an antidepressant. *British Medical Journal* 313(7052):241-242.

22. Johne, A., J. Brockmoller, S. Bauer, A. Maurer, M. Langheinrich, and I. Roots. 1999. Pharmacokinetic interaction of digoxin with an herbal extract from St. John's wort *(Hypericum perforatum). Clinical Pharmacology and Therapeutics.* 66(4):338-345.

23. Ruschitzka, Frank, Peter J. Meier, Marko Turina, Thomas F. Lüscher, and Georg Noll. 2000. Acute heart transplant rejection due to Saint John's wort. *The Lancet* 355:548-549.

24. Piscitelli, Stephen C., Aaron H. Burstein, Doreen Chaitt, Raul M. Alfaro, and Judith Falloon. 2000. Indinavir concentrations and St. John's wort. *The Lancet* 355:547-548.

25. FDA Public Health Advisory. Risk of drug interactions with St. John's wort and indinavir and other drugs. February 10, 2000. <http://www.fda.gov/cder/drug/advisory/stjwort.htm>.

26. Ibid.

27. Suzuki, O., Y. Katsumata, M. Oya, S. Bladt, and H. Wagner. 1984. Inhibition of monamine oxidase by hypericin. *Planta Medica* 50:272-274.

28. Bladt, S., and H. Wagner. 1994. Inhibition of MAO by fractions and constituents of *Hypericum* extract. *Journal of Geriatric Psychiatry and Neurology* 7 (Suppl. 1): S57-S59.

29. De Smet, P.A., and W.A. Nolen. 1996. St. John's wort as an antidepressant. *British Medical Journal* 313:241-247.

30. Muller, W.E., and R. Rossol. 1994. Effects of *Hypericum* extract on the suppression of serotonin receptors. *Journal of Geriatric Psychiatry and Neurology* 7(Suppl. 1):S63-S64.

31. Winterhoff, H. 1993. Pharmacological screening of *Hypericum perforatum* L. in animals. *Nervenheilkunde* 12:341-345.

32. Nathan, P. 1999. The experimental and clinical pharmacology of St. John's Wort (*Hypericum perforatum* L.). *Molecular Psychiatry* 4(4):333-338.

33. Singer, A., M. Wonnemann, and W.E. Muller. 1999. Hyperforin, a major antidepressant constituent of St. John's wort, inhibits serotonin uptake by elevating free intracellular Na^{+1}. *Journal of Pharmacology and Experimental Therapeutics* 290(3):1363-1368.

34. Kaehler, S.T., C. Sinner, S.S. Chatterjee, and A. Philippu. 1999. Hyperforin enhances the extracellular concentrations of catecholamines, serotonin and glutamate in the rat locus coeruleus. *Neuroscience Letters* 262(3):199-202.

35. Firenzuoli, F., and L. Gori. 1999. Is the antidepressant effect of *Hypericum* extracts depending on their hyperforin content? *Forschende Komplementarmedizin* 6(1):27; discussion 27-28.

36. Chatterjee, S.S., M. Noldner, E. Koch, and C. Erdelmeier. 1998. Antidepressant activity of hypericum perforatum and hyperforin: The neglected possibility. *Pharmacopsychiatry* 31(Suppl. 1):7-15.

37. Laakmann, G., C. Schule, T. Baghai, and M. Kieser. 1998. St. John's wort in mild to moderate depression: The relevance of hyperforin for the clinical efficacy. *Pharmacopsychiatry* 31(Suppl. 1):54-59.

38. Muller, W.E., A. Singer, M. Wonnemann, U. Hafner, M. Rolli, and C. Schafer. 1998. Hyperforin represents the neurotransmitter reuptake inhibiting constituent of *Hypericum* extract. *Pharmacopsychiatry* 31(Suppl. 1):16-21.

39. Chatterjee, S.S., S.K. Bhattacharya, M. Wonnemann, A. Singer, and W.E. Muller. 1998. Hyperforin as a possible antidepressant component of *Hypericum* extracts. *Life Sciences* 63(6):499-510.

40. Linde, Klaus, Gilbert Ramirez, Cynthia D. Mulrow, Andrej Pauls, Wolfgang Weidenhammer, and Dieter Melchart. 1996. St. John's wort for depression—An overview and meta-analysis of randomised clinical trials. *British Medical Journal* 313(7052):253-258.

41. *Hypericum* Depression Trial Study Group. 2002. Effect of *Hypericum perforatum* (St. John's Wort) in major depressive disorder: A randomized controlled trial. *Journal of the American Medical Association* 287(14):1807-1814.

42. Ibid, p. 1813.

43. De Feudis, F.V. (Ed.) 1991. *Ginkgo biloba extract (EGb 761): Pharmacological activities and clinical applications.* Paris: Elsevier.

44. Funfgeld, E.W. (Ed.) 1988. *Rokan* (Ginkgo biloba): *Recent results in pharmacology and clinic.* New York: Springer-Verlag.

45. Kleijnen, J., and P. Knipschild. 1992. Ginkgo biloba. *The Lancet* 340:1136-1139.

46. Hofferberth, B. 1994. The efficacy of EGb 761 in patients with senile dementia of the Alzheimer type, a double-blind, placebo-controlled study on different levels of investigation. *Human Psychopharmacology* 9:215-222.

47. Kleijnen, J. 1992. *Ginkgo biloba* for cerebral insufficiency. *British Journal of Clinical Pharmacology* 34(4):352-358.

48. Kanowski, S., W.M. Herrmann, K. Stephan, W. Wierich, and R. Horr. 1997. Proof of the efficacy of the *Ginkgo biloba* special extract EGb 761 in outpatients suffering from mild to moderate primary degenerative dementia of the Alzheimer type of multi-infarct dementia. *Phytomedicine* 4:3-13.

49. Le Bars, Pierre L., Martin M. Katz, Nancy Berman, Turan Itil, Alfred M. Freedman, and Alan F. Schatzberg. 1997. A placebo-controlled, double-blind, randomized trial of an extract of *Ginkgo biloba* for dementia. *Journal of the American Medical Association* 278:1327-1332.

50. Carper, Jean. 1997. Astonishing memory pill (Ginkgo). In *Miracle Cures: Dramatic new scientific discoveries revealing the healing powers of herbs, vitamins, and other natural remedies.* New York: HarperCollins Publishers, p. 64.

51. Ibid, pp. 58-71.

52. Carper, Jean. 1997. Unique infection fighter (Echinacea). In: *Miracle Cures: Dramatic new scientific discoveries revealing the healing powers of herbs, vitamins, and other natural remedies* (pp. 108-119). New York: HarperCollins Publishers.

53. Melchart, D. 1994. Immunodilation with echinacea—a systematic review of controlled clinical trials. *Phytomedicine* 1:245-254.

54. Richman, Alan, and P. Witkowski. Annual herb sales survey. *Whole Foods,* October 2001, pp. 23-30.

55. Bauer, R. 1996. Echinacea drugs—Effects and active ingredients. *Zeitschrift fur Arztliche Fortbildung (Jena)* 90(2):111-115.

56. Bräunig, B., M. Dorn, and E. Knick. 1992. *Echinacea purpurea radix* for strengthening the immune response in flu-like infections. *Zeitschrift Phytotherapie* 13:7-13.

57. Schöneberger, D. 1992. The influence of immune-stimulating effects of pressed juice from *Echinacea purpurea* on the course and severity of colds. *Forum Immunolgie* 8:2-12.

58. Melchart, D., E. Walther, K. Linde, R. Brandmaier, and C. Lersch. 1998. Echinacea root extracts for the prevention of upper respiratory tract infections: A double-blind, placebo-controlled randomized trial. *Archives of Family Medicine* 7(6):541-545.

59. Melchart, D., K. Linde, F. Worku, R. Bauer, and H. Wagner. 1994. Immunomodulation with Echinacea—A systematic review of controlled clinical trials. *Phytomedicine* 1:245-254.

60. Bauer, R. 1996. Echinacea drugs—Effects and active ingredients. *Zeitschrift fur Arztliche Fortbildung* (Jena) 90(2):111-115.

61. McGregor, R.L. 1968. The taxonomy of the genus *Echinacea* (Compositae). *University of Kansas Science Bulletin* 48:113-142.

Chapter 9

1. Food and Drug Administration. 1997. Dietary supplements containing ephedrine alkaloids; proposed rule. *Federal Register* 62(107):30677-30724.

2. General Accounting Office. 1999. Dietary supplements: Uncertainties in analyses underlying FDA's proposed rule on ephedrine alkaloids. Report to the Chairman and Ranking Minority Member, Committee on Science, House of Representatives. GAO/HEHS/GGD-99-90.

3. States push for ephedra restrictions. FDA Hotline. March 1997. *NNFA Today*. April 1997.

4. *Food Labeling and Nutrition News.* May 20, 1998.

5. Herndon, Ray F. Felled by "herbal" diet drug. *Los Angeles Times,* April 4, 2002.

6. Haller, Christine A. and Neal L. Benowitz. 2000. Adverse cardiovascular and central nervous system events associated with dietary supplements containing ephedrine alkaloids. *New England Journal of Medicine* 343(25):1833-1838.

7. Herndon, Ray F. Felled by "herbal" diet drug. *Los Angeles Times,* April 4, 2002.

8. Ibid.

9. Palmer, Mary E. 1999. Problems evaluating contamination of dietary supplements. *New England Journal of Medicine* 340(7):568, Correspondence.

10. Keller, K. 1992. Results of the revision of herbal drugs in the Federal Republic of Germany with a special focus on risk aspects. *Zeitschrift fur Phytotherapie* 116:118.

Chapter 10

1. Eisenberg, David M., Roger B. Davis, Susan L. Ettner, Scott Appel, Sonja Wilkey, Maria Van Rompany, and Ronald C. Kessler. 1998. Trends in alternative medicine use in the United States 1990-1997. *JAMA* 280(18):1569-1575.

2. Brevoort, Peggy. 1998. The booming U.S. botanical market: A new overview. *Herbalgram* 44:33-46.

3. Blumenthal, Mark. 2001. Herb sales up 1% for all channels of trade in 2000. *Herbalgram* 53:63.

4. Dietary Supplement Health and Education Act. 1994. Public Law 103-417, Section 4.

5. Ibid.

6. Office of Inspector General. 2001. Adverse event reporting for dietary supplements: An inadequate safety valve.

7. Commission on Dietary Supplement Labels. 1997. *Report on the Commission on Dietary Supplement Labels,* p. 22.

Chapter 11

1. Manual of Patent Examining Procedure Section 706.03(a): "a thing occurring in nature, which is substantially unaltered, is not a 'manufacture' " and is therefore not patentable matter.

2. Schwabe, Willmar. *Ginkgo biloba:* Important notice. *Natural Business* April 1998.

3. Le Bars, Pierre L., Martin M. Katz, Nancy Berman, Turan Itil, Alfred M. Freedman, and Alan F. Schatzberg. 1997. A placebo-controlled, double-blind, randomized trial of an extract of *Ginkgo biloba* for dementia. *Journal of the American Medical Association* 278:1327-1332.

4. <http://ods.od.nih.gov/grants/botanicals99.html>.

Chapter 12

1. Eisenberg, David M., Roger B. Davis, Susan L. Ettner, Scott Appel, Sonja Wilkey, Maria Van Rompany, and Ronald C. Kessler. 1998. Trends in alternative medicine use in the United States 1990-1997. *JAMA* 280(18):1569-1575.

2. Blendon, R.J., C.M. DesRoches, J.M. Benson, M. Brodie, and D.E. Altman. 2001. Americans' views on the use and regulation of dietary supplements. *Archives of Internal Medicine* 161:805-810 (quote on p. 805).

Chapter 13

1. David A. Kessler in Hearing of the Subcommittee on Health and Environment, Committee on Energy and Commerce, House of Representatives, July 29, 1993.

2. Blendon, R.J., C.M. DesRoches, J.M. Benson, M. Brodie, D.E. Altman. 2001. Americans' views on the use and regulation of dietary supplements. *Archives of Internal Medicine* 161:805-810.

3. Ibid.

4. Commission on Dietary Supplement Labels. 1997. *Report on the Commission on Dietary Supplement Labels,* p. 47.

5. <http://ods.od.nih.gov/databases/ibids.html>.

6. Food and Drug Administration. 1998. Regulations on statements made for dietary supplements concerning the effect of the product on the structure or function of the body. *Federal Register* 63(82):23624-23632 (quote on p. 23627).

7. Dietary Supplement Health and Education Act. 1994. Public Law 103-417, Section 12(c).

8. Commission on Dietary Supplement Labels. 1997. *Report on the Commission on Dietary Supplement Labels,* p. 57.

9. Ibid, p. 54.

10. Ibid, p. 57.

Chapter 14

1. National Institutes of Health, Office of Dietary Supplements, International Bibliographic Information on Dietary Supplements (IBIDS), <http://ods.od.nih.gov/databases/overview_ibids.html>.

2. American Herbal Products Association. 1992. *Herbs of Commerce.*

3. Brevoort, Peggy. 1998. The booming U.S. botanical market: A new overview. *Herbalgram* 44:33-46.

4. Blumenthal, Mark. 1999. Herb market levels after five years of boom: 1999 sales in mainstream market up only 11% in first half of 1999 after 55% increase in 1998. *Herbalgram* 47:64.

5. Blumenthal, Mark. 2001. Herb sales up 1% for all channels of trade in 2000. *Herbalgram* 53:63.

6. Overall supplement sales slightly up. *Natural Products Industry Insider.* March 11, 2002, p. 1.

7. Richman, Alan and P. Witkowski. 2001. Annual herb sales survey. *Whole Foods* October 2001, pp. 23-30.

8. *Nutrition Business Journal.* 1999. *Third Annual Review of the Nutrition Industry* and *Data Book on the Nutrition Industry.*

9. Linde, Klaus, Gilbert Ramirez, Cynthia D. Mulrow, Andrej Pauls, Wolfgang Weidenhammer, and Dieter Melchart. 1996. St. John's wort for depression—An overview and meta-analysis of randomised clinical trials. *British Medical Journal* 313(7052):253-258.

10. Andrews, Edmund L. In Germany, humble herb is a rival to Prozac. *The New York Times.* September 9, 1997, p. C1.

11. Brody, Jane E. Personal Health. *The New York Times.* September 10, 1997, p. C10.

Index

Page numbers followed by the letter "t" indicate tables.